CLINICAL AND LABORATORY MANUAL OF DENTAL IMPLANT ABUTMENTS

CLINICAL AND LABORATORY MANUAL OF DENTAL IMPLANT ABUTMENTS

Edited by

Hamid R. Shafie

Director of Postdoctoral Implant Training, Washington
Hospital Center, Department of Oral and
Maxillofacial Surgery, Washington, DC;
President and Chief Knowledge Officer, American
Institute of Implant Dentistry, Washington, DC;
and Private Practice limited to implant prosthodontics,
Washington, DC

WILEY Blackwell

This edition first published 2014 © 2014 by John Wiley & Sons, Inc.

Editorial offices: 1606 Golden Aspen Drive, Suites 103 and 104, Ames, Iowa 50010, USA
The Atrium, Southern Gate, Chichester, West Sussex, PO19 8SQ, UK
9600 Garsington Road, Oxford, OX4 2DQ, UK

For details of our global editorial offices, for customer services and for information about how to apply for permission to reuse the copyright material in this book please see our website at www.wiley.com/wiley-blackwell.

Library of Congress Cataloging-in-Publication Data
Clinical and laboratory manual of dental implant abutments / edited by Hamid R. Shafie.
     1 online resource.
Includes bibliographical references and index.
   Description based on print version record and CIP data provided by publisher; resource not viewed.
ISBN 978-1-118-92665-9 (Adobe PDF) – ISBN 978-1-118-92853-0 (ePub) – ISBN 978-1-119-94981-7 (hardback)
I. Shafie, Hamid R., editor.
[DNLM: 1. Dental Abutments.   2. Dental Implant-Abutment Design. WU 500]
RK667.I45
617.6'93–dc23

2014024506

A catalogue record for this book is available from the British Library.

Wiley also publishes its books in a variety of electronic formats. Some content that appears in print may not be available in electronic books.

Cover image: courtesy of Mike Chapman

Set in 10/12pt Meridien LT Std by Toppan Best-set Premedia Limited, Hong Kong
Printed and bound in Malaysia by Vivar Printing Sdn Bhd

1   2014

Contents

List of Contributors

Tamer Abdel-Azim, DDS
Assistant Professor,
Department of Oral Health and Rehabilitation,
School of Dentistry,
University of Louisville,
Louisville, KY

Mary L. Ballard, DDS
Oral and Maxillofacial Surgeon,
Private Practice,
Washington, DC

Paul P. Binon, DDS, MSD, FAO
Assistant Research Scientist,
Department of Restorative Dentistry,
University of California at San Francisco,
San Francisco, CA;
Adjunct Professor of Prosthodontics,
Graduate Prosthodontics,
Indiana University,
Indianapolis, IN;
and Private Practice,
Roseville, CA

Robert B. Kerstein, DMD
Former Assistant Clinical Professor,
Department of Restorative Dentistry,
Tufts University School of Dental Medicine,
Boston, MA

Wei-Shao Lin, DDS
Assistant Professor,
Department of Oral Health and Rehabilitation,
School of Dentistry,
University of Louisville,
Louisville, KY

Scott Martyna, DMD
Oral and Maxillofacial Surgery Resident,
Washington Hospital Center,
Department of Oral and Maxillofacial Surgery,
Washington, DC

Dean Morton, BDS, MS
Professor,
Department of Oral Health and Rehabilitation,
School of Dentistry,
University of Louisville,
Louisville, KY

Julian Osorio, DMD, MScD
Assistant Clinical Professor,
Department of Restorative Dentistry,
Tufts University School of Dental Medicine,
Boston, MA

Hamid R. Shafie, DDS, CAGS
Director of Postdoctoral Implant Training,
Washington Hospital Center,
Department of Oral and Maxillofacial Surgery,
Washington, DC;
President and Chief Knowledge Officer,
American Institute of Implant Dentistry, Washington,
   DC;
and Private Practice limited to implant
   prosthodontics,
Washington, DC

Bryan A. White, DMD
Maxillofacial Surgeon,
Private Practice,
Gilbert, AZ

Forewords

With implant dentistry going through such rapid changes over the past few years it is very timely to see a textbook on the latest technology related to implant abutments. Hamid Shafie is to be congratulated for putting together a much needed update of all clinical and laboratory aspects of dental implant abutments. The book is filled with information and references related to different types of abutments, their shapes, the materials used, and the types of connections that are available. In addition, there are chapters on screw technology and abutment materials that are up to date and excellent for both the beginner and the advanced reader. The chapter on CAD-CAM technology is particularly useful as so many clinicians today are using these techniques. The chapters are also filled with excellent diagrams and clinical examples that clearly make the point of the pros and cons of different abutments.

It is a pleasure to see this fine book come to print. It will be a staple in every clinician's and technician's reference library. Congratulations to Dr Shafie and his co-authors for a job well done.

Dennis Tarnow, DDS
Clinical Professor and Director of Implant Dentistry
Columbia University College of Dentistry
New York, NY

The biologic adaptation of soft and hard tissues is omnipotent when considering the surface treatments and the construction of the prosthesis. Platform switching is nicely demonstrated and the Laser-Loc system, to gain optimal collagen attachment to the abutment, is presented. The physical perpendicular attachment of the fibers prevent the apical migration of the epithelium and, thus, offer protection of the crestal bone. Platform switching has been very effective in curtailing the micro-gap issue resulting in the loss of 1.5–2 mm of crestal bone as the result of an inflammatory infiltrate.

This information will simplify a confusing decision where there is a paucity of agreement relative to the selection of abutment. The topic of esthetics is so very important to the patient that it mandates considerable space. The answers are well presented by both text and illustrations and can be converted to optimal patient treatments.

I suggest this book will be of great value to all dentists who seek perfection in their implant endeavors. It should find a place in every office.

Myron Nevins, DDS
Associate Clinical Professor of Periodontology
Harvard School of Dental Medicine
Boston, MA;
Clinical Professor, Department of Periodontics
University of Pennsylvania School of Dental Medicine
Philadelphia, PA;
Clinical Professor, Department of Periodontology
Temple University Kornberg School of Dentistry
Philadelphia, PA;
Former Director and Chairman
American Board of Periodontology
Chicago, IL;
Former President
The American Academy of Periodontology
Chicago, IL

The restorative realm of implant dentistry has become increasingly sophisticated in recent years but simultaneously it has become progressively more complex, complicated and convoluted for the practicing clinician.

Fortunately, Dr. Hamid Shafie has correlated vast amounts of data and information, synthesized it and delivered it to us all in a clinically relevant text. The *Clinical and Laboratory Manual of Dental Implant Abutments* is an invaluable, complete, yet concise text that addresses all aspects of restorative implant dentistry from material selection, through pre-fabricated and custom abutments, and today, the relevance of CAD/CAM manufacturing.

It also covers the key facets of the retaining abutment screw, the biology and mechanics of the different abutment-implant connections, and that consummate evaluative signature of success, the peri-implant soft tissue.

"Digital Dentistry" has had a particularly large impact on the dental implant arena, diagnostically, clinically, and in the rapidly evolving aspect of implant abutments.

3D technologies now facilitate every element of this restorative realm from the diagnosis and initial strategies, through the surgical phases, to the final design and fabrication of the ensuing prosthesis.

This makes the entire implant process easier, more predictable, economically viable, and so available to a greater percentage of the world's population.

Hopefully this text, like Dr. Shafie's previous one, will also be translated into multiple languages and so go on to similarly advance the global clinical possibilities and then reality of implant dentistry for more and more of the world population.

David Garber, DMD
Professor of Departments of Oral Rehabilitation
Medical College of Georgia
Augusta, GA
Clinical Professor in the Department of Prosthodontics
Louisiana State University
Baton Rouge, LA
Clinical Professor in the Department of Restorative Dentistry
University of Texas in San Antonio
Atlanta, GA

Even though sophisticated implant dentistry has been in existence for over a quarter century, the technology continues to advance. The application of implant borne restorations to more diverse and demanding applications has further complicated this field. The emphasis on comprehensive treatment planning including biomechanics, esthetics, and bone maintenance by mechanotransduction, and restorative material attributes, all flow through the myriad of abutment configurations. This comprehensive manual by Dr. Shafie provides an excellent didactic, and visual source of information for every approach and type of implant connection. Importantly it explains material properties

and applications, as well as the biological response to the various configurations and parts. This manual will serve us all as the ultimate guide to decision making, and implementation, of abutment rendered implant prosthetics.

Daniel Spagnoli, DDS MS PhD
Associate Professor & Peltier Chair
Department of Oral & Maxillofacial Surgery
Director of Hospital Affairs
LSU HSC School of Dentistry
New Orleans, LA

There is an increasing need for the oral and maxillofacial surgeon to understand the intricate details of restorative implant dentistry. For the past 10 years, implant manufactures have focused more on design and technology development of abutments than the implant screw itself. CAD/CAM abutments, zirconia abutments, and Laser-Lok™ abutments are a few examples of those advancements. With such a dynamic market, many implant companies are glad to hype the superiority of their different implant abutment connection designs.

Making a crown and cementing it over an abutment is a simple procedure for any dentist. Placing an implant is a simple procedure for any surgeon. The confusion comes from the important intermediate part called the abutment. It is no longer sufficient to just perform precise surgery, since choosing the wrong abutment will most likely lead to implant failure.

While up to now we have had to rely on multiple sources for a discussion on this topic, it is refreshing to find a book that is a concise source of information about implant abutments. This book gives an independent, objective overview of different connection designs and their impact on the crestal bone and eventually on the outcome of treatment. It has the format of a cookbook with lots of illustrations and detailed instructions.

Dr Shafie has considerable experience not just as a prosthodontist but also as an educator of generations of oral and maxillofacial surgery residents in our Department. As a prosthodontist for the past 20 years, he has tried to bridge the gap between surgeons and restorative dentists. The first breakthrough was his overdenture textbook, which was well received globally, and is now complemented by this excellent book following the same vision. In essence, oral surgeons cannot be successful in implant dentistry unless they have full knowledge of the restorative aspects of treatment. Implant dentistry is changing and shifting toward a full service concept. With this perspective, Dr Shafie has produced a unique book of great practicality to oral surgery residents in training as well as to established specialists who want to educate themselves about restorative aspects of implant dentistry.

It is with great pleasure that I recommend this book, which should be essential in the library of all oral surgeons involved in implant dentistry.

George Obeid, DDS
Chairman
Department of Oral and Maxillofacial Surgery
Medstar Washington Hospital Center
Washington, DC

Preface

Almost 40 years after the introduction of osseointegration, and after countless scientific publications by many talented dentists from around the world, I am delighted to present this unique textbook to everybody who is involved in implant dentistry. The subject of implant abutments was previously often simplified and overlooked, or subsumed within bigger clinical subjects and techniques.

A common misunderstanding in implant dentistry is that one type of abutment is suitable in multiple situations. Those who strive for the best implant treatment results for their patients understand that choosing an abutment is not a one-size-fits-all approach. Choosing the correct abutment is integral to achieving a mechanically stable and esthetically pleasing restoration.

This book follows the same format as my first textbook. It is rich with photos, illustrations, and tables. It discusses the details of available abutment materials, types, and components, and gives the clinician the tools to select the appropriate abutment in any clinical situation. Also reviewed are common pitfalls related to abutment choices and failures. All the contributors undertook an extensive literature review to insure each chapter includes the most important references and key articles by other clinicians and scholars.

I had the privilege of working with nine talented clinicians with superior academic backgrounds, who accepted my invitation to share their knowledge and expertise. This book will be a great reference for our colleagues in private practice as it shows step by step how to perform the different treatments. Hopefully educators and key opinion leaders in the field of implant dentistry will also use and recommend this valuable reference to residents and students.

Many thanks to my publisher, Wiley Blackwell, for endless patience, kindness, and most of all giving me encouragement to write another book. I would like to acknowledge and thank my friend and assistant Larisa Zgircha, who coordinated the entire text and images, and Mike Chapman, who is one of the most talented medical illustrators in the dental field and spent countless hours designing the cover of this book to make sure it reflects the heart and soul of what we have written. I cannot thank him enough for his support. Finally, I would like acknowledge all the major implant companies in the world that extended their unconditional support to me and all of the contributors.

Hamid R. Shafie
Washington DC, 2014

Dedications

With love to my wife, Maryam and daughter, Ava for being so understanding and supportive while I was working on this book.

To my parents, Mehdi and Minoo who gave me everything I needed to advance in life.

To my wonderful readers...your positive response to my first book motivated me to write this one. *"Writing a textbook is like a chef preparing a fine dining experience. All of my preparations and efforts are for enjoyment of the readers. Knowing that somebody enjoyed the experience and shared it with others is the best reward for an author."*

To my mentor and friend George Obeid. A man who gave me the best opportunity in my professional life and helped me to realize my dream. I remain grateful forever.

1

Implant Abutment Materials

Hamid R. Shafie[1] and Bryan A. White[2]

[1]Washington Hospital Center, Department of Oral and Maxillofacial Surgery, Washington, DC; and American Institute of Implant Dentistry, Washington, DC
[2]Private Practice, Gilbert, AZ

INTRODUCTION

A wide variety of abutment materials are available on the dental implant market. A major challenge for clinicians today is understanding the biologic response to each material, as well as the best indication for using each of the different types.

To complicate this problem, there are no well defined and comprehensive sources reviewing the properties associated with abutment materials. This chapter provides relevant information on abutment materials and their soft tissue response.

MUCOSAL SEAL

The mucosal seal surrounding a dental implant abutment is an essential factor in preventing bacterial penetration into the crestal bone and around the implant neck. In order to understand the soft tissue response, it is important to be familiar with the anatomy of the mucosal seal.

Natural Dentition

The periodontal soft tissue is an important factor in a person's natural protection against periodontal disease. The biologic width is the depth of soft tissue below the sulcus in the natural dentition. It consists of a junctional epithelium and connective tissue layer. The junctional epithelium ranges from 1 to 2 mm wide followed apically by a 1 mm layer of connective tissue. The alveolar bone lies just below this connective tissue.

In the natural dentition, this zone has been proven to be essential for protecting the periodontium from plaque and bacteria penetration into the oral cavity. The junctional epithelium attaches to the teeth with a hemidesmisomal attachment, providing a shield against bacteria. The connective tissue layer contains collagen fibers that insert into the teeth and cementum perpendicularly to the tooth. These fibers provide additional reinforcement against an apically migrating junctional epithelium caused by periodontal disease.

Peri-implant Mucosal Seal

A mucosal seal surrounding dental implants is also essential in avoiding peri-implantitis. The biologic width surrounding dental implants also contains a junctional epithelium, followed apically by a connective tissue layer. As in the natural dentition, the coronal portion of the biologic width contains the junctional epithelium. In 1984, Gould and colleagues demonstrated that this junctional epithelium attaches to the titanium surface in a similar manner to the natural dentition, with hemidesmosomes. A connective tissue attachment can be found further apically. Buser et al. (1992) described this attachment as being rich in collagen fibers but sparse in cells or resembling scar tissue.

Clinical and Laboratory Manual of Dental Implant Abutments, First Edition. Edited by Hamid R. Shafie.
© 2014 John Wiley & Sons, Inc. Published 2014 by John Wiley & Sons, Inc.

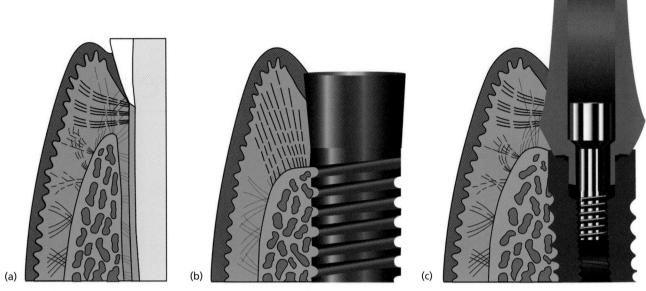

(a)   (b)   (c)

Figure 1.1 Note the perpendicular collagen fibers in the natural dentition (a) and Laser-Lok abutments (c) in comparison to the parallel collagen fibers with other implant abutments (b).

Unlike the natural dentition, in implant abutments the apical connective tissue fibers do not have the same quality of attachments. The natural dentition has dentogingival fibers running perpendicular to the tooth from the bone to the cementum. The connective tissue layer surrounding a dental implant abutment has fibers running in a parallel fashion (Figure 1.1). The only exception to this histology is with Laser-Lok™ abutments which are discussed later in this chapter.

Due to the weakened connective tissue support around implant abutments, the junctional epithelium is believed to be more susceptible to apical migration. In other words, a dental implant is more susceptible to peri-implantitis than a natural tooth is to periodontitis.

It is important to note that this biologic width or "peri-implant seal" protects the implant against peri-implantitis and provides an esthetic result. When considering which abutment type to use one should consider how well the abutment *forms* and *maintains* this mucosal seal.

PELLICLE, BIOFILM, AND PERIODONTAL DISEASE

One of the key factors in selecting an abutment material is its hygienic property. To review the importance of hygiene it is important to understand pellicle formation, subsequent biofilm production, and the pathway of peri-implantitis development.

Pellicle

The process of plaque formation begins with glycoproteins attaching to the surface of the enamel or an abutment, creating a thin layer called the pellicle. Although this layer by itself is harmless, it provides a framework for bacteria to adhere to.

Biofilm

A biofilm is an aggregation of multiple organisms coexisting together. Initially, Gram-positive aerobic cocci adhere to this thin glycoprotein layer or pellicle. As these bacteria multiply, the bacterial colonies multiply creating a more anaerobic environment. This anaerobic environment then permits more harmful Gram-negative rods to collect within the biofilm. The biofilm creates an acidic environment that contributes to dental caries but, more relevant to the topic at hand, the biofilm also contributes to periodontal disease.

Periodontal Disease in the Natural Dentition

Periodontal disease is caused by the biofilm, which destroys the periodontium and causes loss of the alveolar bone and inflammation of the periodontal tissues. This is not a novel development – the landmark paper by Page and Schroeder outlined this process of periodontal disease back in 1976.

Peri-implantitis

As in the natural dentition, development of the pellicle and biofilm and subsequent inflammation also occurs with dental implants. This process can cause the potential for apical migration of the peri-implant seal and bone loss. The process of peri-implantitis is more common with dental implants than periodontal disease is with natural dentition. This is because the peri-implant mucosal seal is not as effective (except in the case of Laser-Lok abutments) as the mucosal seal surrounding the natural dentition.

As will be discussed, some abutments have enhanced capabilities for resisting bacterial colonization. Other abutments have improved capabilities for forming a more resistant mucosal seal with a strengthened connective tissue attachment.

IMPLANT ABUTMENT MATERIAL RELATED RESEARCH

The remainder of this chapter focuses on the variety of abutments available on the market. Different abutment materials will be compared in terms of their ability to *form* and *maintain* the "peri-implant seal." Carefully chosen research has been selected to demonstrate how the varieties of abutments specifically affect soft tissue.

The most commonly used implant abutment materials (Figure 1.2, Table 1.1) to be discussed are:

- Titanium:
  - machined
  - polished
  - Laser-Lok.
- Surgical grade stainless steel.
- Cast gold.
- Zirconia.
- Polyether ether ketone (PEEK).

Titanium

Physical properties

Titanium is the only element that offers the unique combination of strength, light weight, and biocompatibility, as well as being extremely durable and strong. Titanium has high corrosion resistant and the highest strength to weight ratio of any known element (Figure 1.3).

Titanium abutments are either made of commercially pure titanium or titanium alloy.

Commercially pure titanium Commercially pure (CP) titanium is widely utilized for medical applications

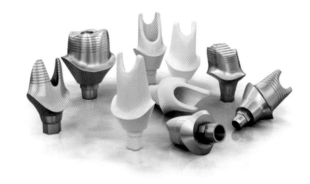

Figure 1.2 Different types of abutments made of different materials by Dentsply Implants.

Table 1.1 Abutment materials and soft tissue response

Abutment material	Forming the peri-implant seal	Maintaining the peri-implant seal
Titanium (machined or polished)	Long-term studies supporting favorable soft tissue results with machined or polished titanium. Most validated abutment material in the literature	Long-term studies supporting favorable soft tissue maintenance with machined or polished titanium. Most validated abutment material in the literature
Titanium abutments with a Laser-Lok transmucosal collar	Greatest ability to form a connective tissue attachment compared with all other abutment materials on the market	Strongest peri-implant seal permitting improved long-term soft tissue maintenance (comparable mucosal seal to the natural dentition)
Gold	Conflicting studies in the literature concerning the ability to form an adequate peri-implant seal	Conflicting studies concerning the long-term maintenance of the peri-implant seal
PEEK (polyether ether ketone)	Comparable soft tissue results to titanium	Comparable hygienic properties to titanium
Zirconia	Comparable ability to form a peri-implant seal to that of machined or polished titanium	Most hygienic abutment on the market allowing improved long-term maintenance of the peri-implant seal

because of its corrosion resistant, high strength, and biocompatible applications. The mechanical properties of CP titanium are influenced by small additions of oxygen and iron. By careful control of these additions, the various grades of CP titanium are produced to give properties suited to different applications. CP titanium with the lowest oxygen and iron levels makes the most formable grade of material; while progressively higher oxygen content results in higher strength levels.

Commercially pure titanium grades

- CP titanium grade 1 (*softest*)
- CP titanium grade 2
- CP titanium grade 3
- CP titanium grade 4 (*hardest*)

Color   Titanium abutments come either with a silver gold color coating (Figure 1.4).

The gold color coating over the surface of the abutment is called titanium nitride. The titanium nitride (TiN; sometimes known as "Tinite," "TiNite," or "TiN") coating is created by a plasma coating process in which titanium and nitrogen ions are combined with TiN, and then molecularly bonded with the titanium substrate of the abutment. TiN was first used in the medical device industry in the 1980s. Biocompatibility testing has been conducted on TiN over many years and this testing, as well as subsequent clinical applications, has demonstrated that TiN is biocompatible and appropriate for use in implantable medical devices that come in contact with bone, skin, tissues, or blood (Figure 1.5).

Titanium nitride is an extremely hard ceramic material, often used as a coating over the titanium component to not only improve the substrate's surface properties but also to achieve a warm, esthetic tone under the gingiva because of its gold shaded hue. Generally, the TiN coating covers the entire abutment except for the contact area between the abutment/implant and screw/abutment. This type of titanium abutment is ideal for esthetically challenging cases with thin soft tissue or when using an all-ceramic crown. In most applications the TiN coating is less than 5 micrometers (0.00020 inches) thick. This coating is only meaningful with CAD/CAM milled abutments where the abutment is not adjusted. Prefabricated abutments are adjusted and generally will lose any strength added by the nitrates following the abutment adjustment.

Titanium alloy (Ti-6Al-4V, Ti6Al4V, or Ti-6-4)

Titanium alloy is also called grade 5 titanium. Titanium alloy contains 6% aluminum, 4% vanadium, 0.25% (maximum) iron, 0.2% (maximum) oxygen, and the remainder titanium. Ti-6Al-4V alloy is significantly stronger than commercially pure titanium and offers better tensile strength and fracture resistance (Figure 1.6).

Because of titanium's unique physical properties, titanium abutments are the first choice for posterior implants. These abutments are available as prefabricated stock or CAD/CAM milled customized abutments.

There is an extensive literature validating the favorable soft tissue response with titanium abutments. Because the majority of the research about peri-implant tissue and abutment materials is based on titanium abutment, this material has become a reference point in describing the properties of other abutment materials.

Machined versus polished titanium and soft tissue responses

Surface roughness is the key difference between machined and polished titanium. This section evaluates whether there is a clinically significant difference between the soft tissue response to polished and machined titanium.

The break down of the peri-implant seal is brought on by the development of a pellicle, biofilm, and inflammation followed by alveolar bone loss. It is well established that the initial glycoproteins and biofilm are more likely to attach to a rough surface than a smooth one. With this logic it could be wrongly assumed that abutments with a smoother surface have less inflammatory response, thus less bone resorption. However, multiple clinical studies have failed to show a clinically significant relationship between an inflammatory response and a roughened abutment surface.

To provide one of many examples, Zitzmann's study concluded that there was no relation between inflammatory response and the abutment surface roughness (Abrahamsson et al. 2002).

Zitzmann's study on the differences in soft tissue response with smooth and rough abutments

- This study used four implants into the premolar regions of five separate beagle dogs
- After 3 months abutments roughened with acid etching and smoother abutments with a turned surface characteristic were placed
- Six months later biopsies of the implants and the surrounding soft and hard tissues were obtained
- No significant differences were noted between the soft tissue attachments near the rough and smooth abutments

In conclusion, although it has been shown that bacteria are more likely to aggregate on a roughened surface, clinical studies between titanium abutments on the market fail to show this relationship. There is no clinically significant different soft tissue response to machined and polished titanium.

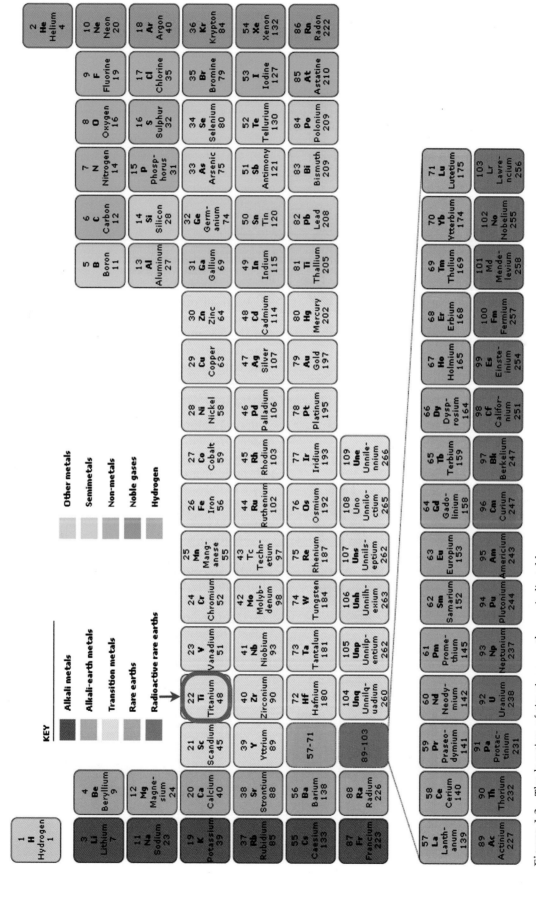

Figure 1.3   The location of titanium on the periodic table.

Prefabricated abutments with a Laser-Lok surface characteristic are a new innovative product (Figure 1.7). The Laser-Lok consists of 8–12 micron titanium micro-channels. These micro-channels provide the following advantages:

- They enhance the establishment of a connective tissue attachment.
- They inhibit the apical migration of the junctional epithelium.
- They preserve the crestal bone.

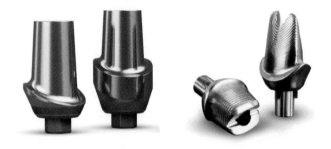

Figure 1.4   Gold (left) and silver (right) color titanium abutments.

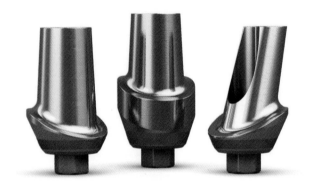

Figure 1.5   Titanium nitride abutments.

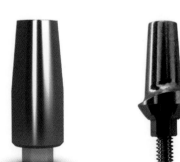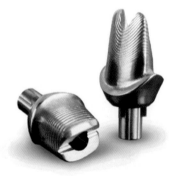

Figure 1.6   Silver titanium alloy abutments.

> **Nevins et al.'s study on soft tissue healing using Laser-Lok**
>
> - A prospective preclinical trial using a canine model to compare Laser-Lok abutments to machined titanium abutment surfaces
> - The study confirmed that the Laser-Lok abutments inhibited the apical migration of the junctional epithelium, prevented coronal resorption, and provided a connective tissue attachment
> - On histologic examination the Laser-Lok design provided healing in a similar fashion to the natural dentition. The connective tissue fibers healed perpendicular to the abutment surface demonstrating the rationale behind Laser-Lok's favorable soft tissue maintenance

With all other implant abutments on the market, connective tissue forms in a weakened parallel fashion to the abutment. The Laser-Lok technology enables the formation of an improved mucosal seal similar to the natural dentition, thus giving it a bright future.

Surgical Grade Stainless Steel

Surgical stainless steel is a specific type of stainless steel used in medical applications, and includes alloying elements of chromium, nickel, and molybdenum. The chromium gives the metal its scratch resistance and corrosion resistance. The nickel provides a smooth and polished finish. The molybdenum gives greater hardness and helps maintain a cutting edge.

Stainless steel is easy to clean and sterilize, strong, and corrosion resistant. Nickel/chrome/molybdenum alloys are sometimes used for implant abutments, but immune system reaction to nickel is a potential complication. Surgical grade stainless steel can be used for temporary implant abutments but is not an ideal material of choice for permanent implant abutment.

Cast Gold

Implant manufacturers recognized the limitations of early "stock abutments" and developed a castable abutment called a UCLA abutment. This abutment is comprised of a machined-fit gold alloy base that fits to the corresponding implant head, combined with a plastic sleeve which can be cut, modified, and added to with wax prior to casting into gold (Figure 1.8).

Cast gold abutments were used to fabricate implant-level, custom-cast restorations that provided subgingi-val margins for esthetics, reduced height for vertical occlusal clearance, and/or custom angles. Cast gold abutments were popular during 1980s and 1990s but with the introduction of more sophisticated stock abutments and CAD/CAM milled abutments they have lost popularity.

- *Gold specs:* 60–65% gold, 20–25% palladium, 19% platinum, and 1% iridium (not a ceramic alloy).
- *Melting range:* Solid, 1400°C; liquid, 1490°C.
- *Recommended casting alloys:* High palladium or high noble porcelain fusing alloys or type III or type IV high noble dental alloys.

Generally, a plastic UCLA abutment is waxed up and customized to an ideal geometry and shape. After investing, the wax and plastic UCLA are burned out of the pattern following the lost wax process. When molten alloy is cast into the investment mold, the gold base component of the UCLA abutment is incorporated into the casting and provides a machined interface that precisely fits the implant. The gold base is fabricated from a non-oxidizing alloy that promotes chemical adhesion of the cast alloy, but does not permit the adhesion of porcelain.

Relevant Studies Comparing Gold, Porcelain, Titanium, and Aluminum

Since the late 1990s there has been a consensus that gold and porcelain have a worse soft tissue response

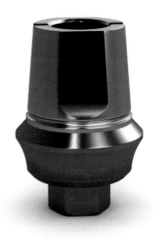

Figure 1.7   Laser-Lok abutment. Courtesy of BioHorizons.

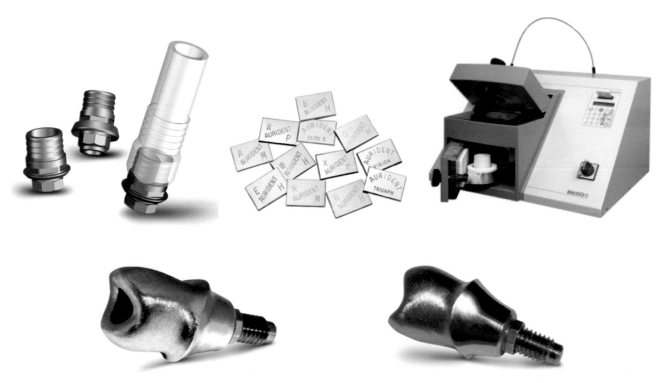

Figure 1.8   Cast gold abutment.

in comparison with aluminum oxide (an outdated ceramic material) and titanium. Much of this thought process comes from Abrahamsson et al.'s 1998 animal study. As a result of this study many clinicians have avoided gold and porcelain abutments altogether.

Abrahamsson et al.'s study comparing the use of titanium and aluminum with gold and porcelain

- Five beagle dogs were used for dental implantation
- Each dog had two commercially pure titanium abutments, two aluminum oxide abutments, one short titanium abutment with attached porcelain fused to gold, and one gold abutment placed
- After 6 months the titanium and aluminum oxide abutments had formed a junctional epithelium of 2 mm and a connective tissue portion of 1–1.5 mm in height
- After 6 months the gold and porcelain abutments had no attachment formed at the abutment level. The soft tissue margin had receded and the bone resorbed
- It was concluded that titanium and aluminum oxide abutments have a favorable soft tissue response over gold or porcelain

Rompen's 2006 literature review agreed with Abrahamsson's findings. Rompen concluded that titanium, aluminum, and zirconia were found to have favorable long-term biocompatibility with soft tissue where gold and porcelain were shown to be less biocompatible.

Abrahamsson and Rompen's conclusions have faced challenges by other studies. The most notable conflicting study is a human study by Vigolo et al. in 2006. They concluded that there was not a significant difference in peri-implant marginal bone and soft tissue response when titanium or gold alloy abutments are used.

Vigolo et al.'s study on soft tissue response to gold and titanium

- 20 single-tooth bilateral edentulous patients (utilizing 40 implants) were used in the trial
- One side of the arch was restored using a gold abutment while the contralateral side was restored using a titanium abutment
- Four years after prosthetic restoration the bilateral sites were examined for supragingival plaque, gingival inflammation, bleeding on probing, the amount of keratinized gingiva, and probing depth
- No significant differences were found in the peri-implant marginal bone levels or soft tissue responses

Vigolo determined that if only the soft tissue response is considered, the choice between using a gold or titanium abutment is merely up to clinician preference. The gold and the titanium were shown to form and maintain an appropriate soft tissue response within this human study.

In addition, Abrahamsson's work with Cardaropoli in 2007 contradicted his earlier findings. In this study Abrahamsson utilized one-piece implants in beagle dogs where the transmucosal portion of the implants were made of gold or titanium. No significant soft tissue differences were found while utilizing titanium or gold at the transmucosal tissue level. However, Abrahamson's work with Welander the next year (Welander et al. 2008) established again that titanium and zirconia had a superior soft tissue result in comparison to gold.

Studies concerning gold abutments have been conflicting. It is difficult to assess where the inconsistencies stem from. However, a few significant disadvantages with gold should be mentioned.

First, titanium and zirconia have the benefit of utilizing CAD/CAM milled technology. With CAD/CAM every abutment is consistent because the CAD/CAM milling machine removes the human element from creating an abutment. Gold abutments are cast in a lab by a technician. One possible explanation for the variable soft tissue response found in studies may be attributed to the expertise of the lab technician. Another issue that arises with gold abutments is sterility. Titanium and zirconia abutments are consistently sterile prior to placement. Gold abutments, after fabrication in a lab, may have inconsistencies with sterility prior to placement.

Zirconia

Zirconium dioxide (ZrO_2), also known as *zirconia* (not to be confused with zircon), is a white crystalline oxide of zirconium. Its most naturally occurring form, with a monoclinic crystalline structure, is the mineral baddeleyite.

Baddeleyite is a rare zirconium oxide mineral (ZrO_2 or zirconia), occurring in a variety of monoclinic prismatic crystal forms. It is transparent to translucent, has high indices of refraction, and ranges from colorless to yellow, green, and dark brown (Figure 1.9). Baddeleyite is a refractory mineral, with a melting point of 2700°C.

Advances in biomaterial science and ceramic manufacturing technology have allowed the production of high strength and biocompatible zirconia that can be used in biomedical devices and implant abutments. The introduction of yettria partially stabilized tetragonal zirconia polycrystals (Y-TZP), powder injection molding (PIM), and hot isostatic pressing (HIP) tech-

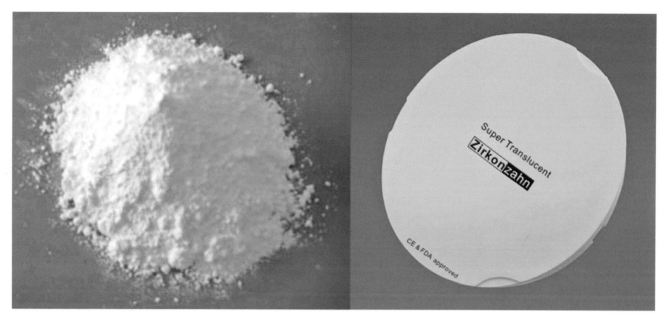

Figure 1.9 Zirconia powder (left) and blank (right).

niques were the hallmarks of this development. Other developments such as the use of zirconia-toughened alumina and ceria-doped zirconia to minimize the incidence and halt the progression of zirconia aging are also considered as key steps in the growing popularity of zirconia as a bioceramic.

Because of its material properties and strength, zirconia is utilized whenever esthetic considerations are important and high loads are expected (e.g. esthetic zone cases, posterior fixed prosthesis frameworks, implant abutments, and multi-unit implant restorations). Zirconia has a high bending strength and fracture toughness, and a Young's modulus comparable to that of steel. In addition to its strength, the greatest advantage of ZrO_2 is its excellent tissue integration. Various studies have demonstrated the successful application of zirconia abutments in terms of stability of soft tissue and marginal bone. Results indicate that the type of material used affects both the amount and quality of the surrounding tissues (when comparing zirconia with cast gold alloys). Also, ziconia abutments minimize bacterial and plaque adhesion and prevent soft tissue inflammation.

Because of its physical properties, adjustment and grinding can be challenging for dentists and dental technicians. Post-sintering adjustment of zirconia components significantly increases the risk of micro-cracks that could result in subsequent failure under clinical function.

Physical properties

ZrO_2 adopts a monoclinic crystal structure at room temperature and transitions to tetrgonal and cubic structures at higher temperatures. The volume expansion caused by the cubic to tetragonal to monoclinic transformation induces large stresses, and these stresses cause ZrO_2 to crack upon cooling from high temperatures. When the ziconia is blended with some other oxides such as yttrium oxide (Y_2O_3, yttria), the tetragonal and/or cubic phases are stabilized (Figure 1.10).

Even though different brands of zirconia can be chemically similar they are not necessarily the same. Different brands of zirconia ceramic are chemically similar, but once processed it can exhibit different mechanical and optical characteristics. When working with zirconia there are differences in machinability (e.g. wet milling and dry milling) and in sintering (e.g. sintering temperature for Vita™ YZ-Cube is 1530°C; for Lava™ frameworks is 1500°C; for Cercon™ is 1350°C).

What is different? In principle, there is pre-sintered zirconia and HIP zirconia available on the market. The pre-sintered zirconia is milled and the material still has a soft, chalk-like consistency (Figure 1.11). For full density, it is sintered again after milling. HIP material is milled in the fully sintered state (Figure 1.12). Note that the processing parameters for pre-sintered zirconia affect its performance attributes.

Pre-sintered zirconia is prepared by three main steps (Figure 1.13). The zirconia powder is pressed and pre-sintered. This is usually done by the manufacturer. The dental lab mills the pre-sintered blank and then sinters the coping or framework to achieve full density. Preparation of the pre-sintered blanks by the manufacturer differs depending on the zirconia powder source and both the pressing and the pre-sintering conditions selected.

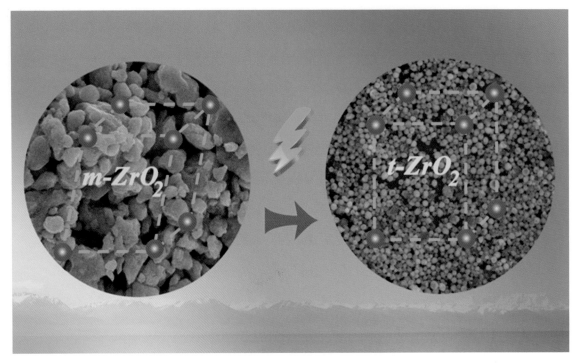

Figure 1.10 Structural differences between monocline and tetragonal zirconia. Courtesy of Professor Naoto Koshizaki, reproduced with permission.

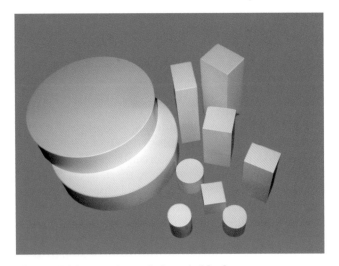

Figure 1.11 Pre-sintered zirconia blank.

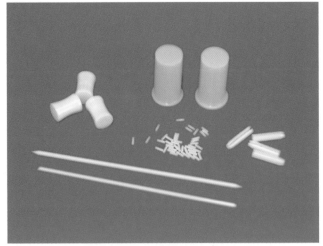

Figure 1.12 HIP-sintered blanks.

1. *Powder.* The available zirconia powders can have different grain sizes, different distributions of the various grain sizes, and different additives (e.g. binder for the pressing step). The additives yttrium oxide and alumina can be distributed within the material in a variety of ways, such as a homogene-ous distribution throughout the whole material, higher concentration at grain borders, etc. The grain size has an effect on strength and transforma-tion toughening – a special and key mechanical characteristic of zirconia. Variations in grain size distribution affect the resulting porosity and hence

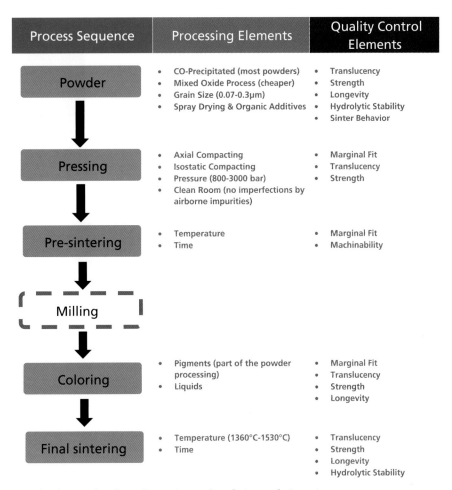

Figure 1.13 Main steps in the production of pre-sintered and sintered zirconia.

the translucency of the material. The distribution of additives can affect the hydrothermal stability of the sintered material.

Note: Differences in the zirconia powder affect the strength/long-term stability and translucency of the abutment.

2. *Pressing conditions*. The powder is first pressed, which can be accomplished by different procedures (e.g. isostatically or axially). The pressing conditions are adjusted to get an optimized blank for the pre-sintering step. The pressing methodology influences the homogeneity and the density distribution of the material and hence the marginal fit. The pressing conditions can lead to differences in strength and translucency and affect the final sintering temperature of the zirconia.

Note: The pressing condition and pressing method affect the marginal fit, strength, and translucency of the restoration.

3. *Pre-sintering*. The pressed zirconia powder is then pre-sintered in a furnace with an optimized temperature profile to generate a blank with suitable strength and millability.

Note: Pre-sintering conditions affect the strength of the pre-sintered material and its millability.

4. *Coloring*. Some zirconia materials can be colored in the pre-sintered state by immersing the copings, abutments, and frameworks in a dyeing liquid. This enables the absorption of coloring agents in the zirconia material. Coloring can be achieved either by pigments (grains) or non-pigmented (ions) agents. It is important to control the effect of the dyeing liquid on the mechanical characteristics of the zirconia material (Figure 1.14).

Note: Coloring of the zirconia can affect the marginal fit, strength, and translucency of the material.

In summary, the zirconia used in dentistry is chemically similar but not necessarily alike.

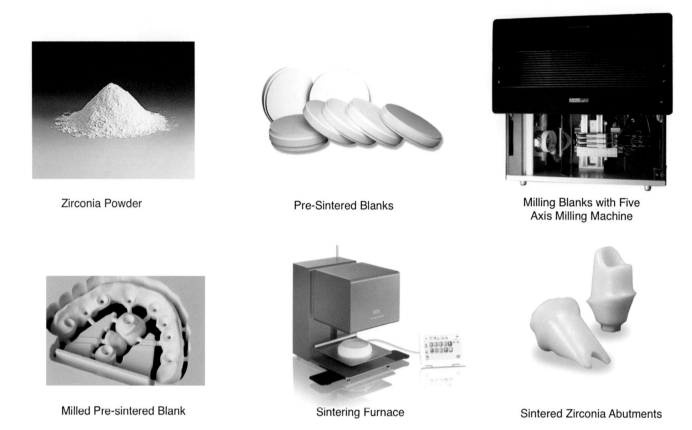

Zirconia Powder

Pre-Sintered Blanks

Milling Blanks with Five Axis Milling Machine

Milled Pre-sintered Blank

Sintering Furnace

Sintered Zirconia Abutments

Figure 1.14   Process of making zirconia abutment from pre-sintered zirconia.

Table 1.2   Comparison of the physical properties of different dental implant materials

	Titanium alloy grade 5	CPT4	Zirconia	Bone
Tensile strength (MPA)	993	662	1000	104–121
Compressive strength (MPA)	970	328	2000	170
Modules of elasticity (GPA)	113.8	103	200	10–15

CPT4, commercially pure titanium grade 4.

Table 1.2 provides a comparative analysis of zirconia's physical properties to bone, commercially pure titanium, and titanium alloy.

These physical properties present adjustment and grinding challenges to dentists and dental technicians. Post-sintering adjustment of zirconia components significantly increases the risk of micro-cracks that could result in subsequent failure during clinical use.

In addition to its strength, the greatest advantage of ZrO_2 is its excellent tissue integration. Various studies have demonstrated the successful application of zirconia abutments in terms of soft tissue and crestal bone stability. Zirconia abutments provide a less plaque-retentive environment around a final prosthesis compared with any other type of abutment material. This improves a patient's ability to maintain a higher level of oral hygiene around the final prosthesis.

Sample studies on the hygenic properties of zirconia

Studies have demonstrated that zirconia has a lower bacterial count and inflammatory infiltrate compared with titanium. Because of zirconia's hygienic properties it has natural benefits in maintaining esthetic soft tissue and preserving crestal bone.

Rimondini et al. performed in vitro and in vivo tests comparing bacteria accumulation on zirconia and titanium. They concluded that zirconia accumulated fewer bacteria than titanium.

Rimondini et al.'s study on the hygienic properties of zirconia compared with titanium

In vitro test
- Disks of titanium and zirconia were used and tested for bacteria accumulation
- Cultures were incubated for 4 days and the bacterial counts were measured
- Zirconia showed significantly less bacterial growth

In vivo test
- Zirconia and titanium were placed onto silicone stents and attached to orthodontic wires intraorally
- The stents were worn for 24 hours and removed
- Bacterial counts were measured on the zirconia and titanium
- Zirconia was found to have a lower bacterial count than the titanium

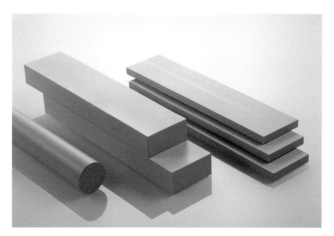

Figure 1.15 PEEK blanks.

Scarano et al.'s 2004 work also aimed at comparing the hygienic properties of titanium and zirconia. Their results were similar to Rimondini's results – that zirconia is a more hygienic material.

Poortinga et al.'s 1999 research demonstrated that zirconia's resistance to bacterial adhesion is likely due to the electron conductivity of this material. They demonstrated that the charge transfer occurs during bacterial adhesion. Bacteria that donate electrons adhere to the substrate more strongly than bacteria that accept electrons.

Inflammatory response with zirconia use

A natural response to the presence of bacteria is the release of inflammatory mediators which leads to bone loss. Rather than evaluating the biofilm, another method of evaluating hygienic properties is to evaluate inflammatory factors such as vascular endothial growth factor (VEGF), nitric oxide synthase expression, inflammatory infiltrate, and microvessel density in the peri-implant soft tissues. An increased level of these factors indicates the presence of inflammation due to bacteria accumulation.

In 2006, Degidi et al. used these inflammatory markers to evaluate the hygienic properties of zirconia compared with titanium.

Degidi et al.'s study on inflammatory infiltrate levels with zirconia and titanium

- Implants were placed into human patients
- Half of the abutments were made of zirconia, while the other half were titanium abutments
- After 6 months biopsies were taken and analyzed for inflammatory mediators
- Significantly less inflammatory infiltrate was noted around the zirconia abutments compared with the titanium abutments

As a side note, regardless of the material used, if there is a micro-gap between the implant and abutment, inflammation and crestal bone loss may occur. As a result, platform switching has been proposed as a solution to reduce the gap and limit crestal bone loss.

Polyether Ether Ketone (PEEK)

PEEK has become the most popular material for fabricating temporary abutment. It is a beige or white colored organic polymer and a semicrystalline thermoplastic with excellent mechanical and chemical resistance properties. The Young's modulus is 3.6 GPa and its tensile strength 90–100 MPa. PEEK has a glass transition temperatures at around 143°C and melts at around 343°C (662°F). It is highly resistant to thermal degradation as well as attack by both organic elements and moist environments. These robust properties have made PEEK an ideal material for temporary abutment (Figure 1.15).

Technical advantages

- Ability to be sterilized without degradation in mechanical properties or biocompatibility.
- Compatibility with X-ray, magnetic resonance imaging (MRI), and computed tomography (CT) imaging without producing artifacts.
- Excellent mechanical properties such as stiffness and durability.
- High compressive strength.
- Proven hard and soft tissue biocompatibility.
- Natural color for excellent aesthetics (Figure 1.16).
- Metal-free solution eliminates ions exchange in the mouth.
- Ease of chairside preparation and modification by dentists.

As early as 1987, Williams et al. provided an animal study demonstrating that PEEK was biocompatible.

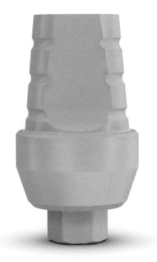

Figure 1.16   PEEK abutment.

Hunter and colleagues, in 1995, compared PEEK with titanium and cobalt chromium (CoCr) for orthopedic uses. They did not note any difference between fibroblastic or osteoblastic attachments with PEEK and those with titanium or CoCr.

Within dentistry, PEEK polymers are used to manufacture restorative and healing abutments. Unlike the orthopedic literature, dental implant research concerning PEEK polymers is limited but what is available is promising.

Koutouzis et al., in 2011, provided a human prospective study comparing titanium and PEEK healing abutments. It was concluded that after 3 months there was not a significant difference between the two materials in terms of soft and hard tissue response. The response was measured in terms of plaque, bleeding on probing, and gingival and crestal bone height.

Another study by Volpe et al., in 2008, compared PEEK with titanium healing abutments using real-time polymerase chain reaction (PCR) in terms of bacterial colonization. After 2 weeks following second stage surgery, no statistical differences were noted between titanium and PEEK abutments in terms of bacterial colonization.

For provisional restorative abutments or healing abutments, PEEK abutments are the first-line option.

CONCLUSIONS

- *Titanium abutments:* There is an extensive literature showing there should be no reservations concerning the use of titanium abutments. Due to the strength of titanium implants they should be considered as the first choice for posterior implants.

- *Machined versus polished titanium abutments:* The commercially available titanium abutments are not significantly different enough from one another to have a clinical impact. Clinically, the surface roughness of the dental abutments on the market is a non-issue.

- *Laser-Lok titanium abutments:* Laser-Lok titanium abutments are superior to titanium abutments without a Laser-Lok transmucosal portion in all clinical scenarios. They are highly recommended in anterior esthetic cases or with patients who have a thin gingival biotype.

- *Stainless steel abutments:* Since the immune systems reacts to the nickel in stainless steel there is a potential complication if it used as a permanent abutment. Surgical grade stainless steel can be used for temporary implant abutments in the short term only.

- *Gold abutments:* Due to contradictory research, clinically it would be prudent to use gold abutments cautiously. In anterior esthetic cases, patients with thin gingiva, or other clinically sensitive cases one should consider another abutment option until more definitive research is available.

- *Zirconia abutments:* Zirconia is the most hygienic abutment on the market and maintains the mucosal seal better than titanium. It is highly recommend for anterior esthetic cases, for patients with thin gingiva, and for any patient with questionable oral hygiene (e.g. with an overdenture where an elderly patient may lack dexterity).

- *PEEK abutments:* When used as a temporary restorative abutment, a clinician should expect a similar soft tissue response as seen with the use of titanium. PEEK abutments are the first line choice for temporary abutments.

REFERENCES AND ADDITIONAL READING

Abrahamsson, I. & Cardaropoli, G. (2007). Peri-implant hard and soft tissue integration to dental implants made of titanium and gold. *Clinical Oral Implants Research*, 18(3), 269–274.

Abrahamsson, I., Berglundh, T., Glantz, P., & Lindhe, J. (1998). The mucosal attachment at different abutments. An experimental study in dogs. *Journal of Clinical Periodontology*, 25(9), 721–727.

Abrahamsson, I., Zitzmann, N.U., Berglundh, T., Linder, E., Wennerberg, A., & Lindhe, J. (2002). The mucosal attachment to titanium implants with different surface characteristics: an experimental study in dogs. *Journal of Clinical Periodontology*, 29(5), 448–455.

Adatia, N.D., Bayne, S.C., Cooper, L.F., & Thompson, J.Y. (2009). Fracture resistance of yttria-stabilized zirconia dental implant abutments. *Journal of Prosthodontics*, 18(1), 17–22.

Aherne, T., & Aherne, S. (2008). Zirconia abutment for the single tooth implant. *Implant Practice*, 1(1), 60–65.

Andersson, B., Glauser, R., Maglione, M., & Taylor, A. (2003). Ceramic implant abutments for short-span FPDs: a prospective 5-year multicenter study. *International Journal of Prosthodontics*, 16(6), 640–646.

Andreiotelli, M., Wenz, H.J., & Kohal, R. (2009). Are ceramic implants a viable alternative to titanium implants? A systematic literature review. *Clinical Oral Implants Research*, 20, 32–47.

Artzi, Z., Tal, H., Moses, O., & Kozlovsky, A. (1993). Mucosal considerations for osseointegrated implants. *Journal of Prosthetic Dentistry*, 70(5), 427–432.

Att, W., Kurun, S., Gerds, T., & Strub, J. (2006). Fracture resistance of single-tooth implant-supported all-ceramic restorations: an in vitro study. *Journal of Prosthetic Dentistry*, 95(2), 111–116.

Berglundh, T., Lindhe, J., Marinell, C., Ericsson, I., & Liljenberg, B. (1992). Soft tissue reaction to de novo plaque formation on implants and teeth. An experimental study in the dog. *Clinical Oral Implants Research*, 3(1), 1–8.

Bollen, C. & Quirynen, M. (1998). The evolution of the surface roughness of different oral hard materials in comparison to the "threshold surface roughness." A review of the literature. *Journal of Dental Materials*, 13(4), 258–269.

Bollen, C.L., Papaioanno, W., Van Eldere, J., Schepers, E., Quirynen, M., & Van Steenberghe, D. (1996). The influence of abutment surface roughness on plaque accumulation and peri-implant mucositis. *Clinical Oral Implants Research*, 7(3), 201–211.

Broggini, N., McManus, L., Hermann, J., et al. (2003). Persistent acute inflammation at the implant–abutment interface. *Journal of Dental Research*, 82(3), 232–237.

Buser, D., Weber, H.P., Donath, K., Fiorellini, J.P., Paquette, D.W., & Williams, R.C. (1992). Soft tissue reactions to non-submerged unloaded titanium implants in beagle dogs. *Journal of Periodontology*, 63(3), 225–35

Butz, F., Heydecke, G., Okutan, M., & Strub, J.R. (2005). Survival rate, fracture strength and failure mode of ceramic implant abutments after chewing simulation. *Journal of Oral Rehabilitation*, 32(11), 838–843.

Degidi, M., Artese, L., Scarano, A., Perrotti, V., Gehrke, P., & Piattelli, A. (2006). Inflammatory infiltrate, microvessel density, nitric oxide synthase expression, vascular endothelial growth factor expression, and proliferative activity in peri-implant soft tissues around titanium and zirconium oxide healing caps. *Journal of Periodontology*, 77(1), 73–80.

Glauser, R., Sailer, I., Wohlwend, A., Studer, S., Schibli, M., & Schärer, P. (2004). Experimental zirconia abutments for implant-supported single-tooth restorations in esthetically demanding regions: 4-year results of a prospective clinical study. *International Journal of Prosthodontics*, 17(3), 285–290.

Gomes, A. & Montero, J. (2011). Zirconia implant abutments: a review. *Medicina Oral Patologia Oral Y Cirugia Bucal*, 16(1), e50–55.

Gould, T.R., Westbury, L., & Brunette, D.M. (1984). Ultrastructural study of the attachment of human gingiva to titanium in vivo. *Journal of Prosthetic Dentistry*, 52, 418–420.

Hunter, A., Archer, C.W., Walker, P.S., & Blunn, G.W. (1995). Attachment and proliferation of osteoblasts and fibroblasts on biomaterials for orthopaedic use. *Biomaterials*, 16(4), 287e95.

Kohal, R., Att, W., Bächle, M., & Butz, F. (2008). Ceramic abutments and ceramic oral implants. An update. *Periodontology 2000*, 47(1), 224–243.

Koutouzis, T., Richardson, J., & Lundgren, T. (2011). Comparative soft and hard tissue responses to titanium and polymer healing abutments. *Journal of Oral Implantology*, 37(1), 174–182.

Linkevicius, T., Apse, P., & Pros, D. (2008). Influence of abutment material on stability of peri-implant tissues: a systematic review. *International Journal of Oral and Maxillofacial Implants*, 23, 449–456.

Manicone, P., Rossiiommetti, P., & Raffaelli, L. (2007). An overview of zirconia ceramics: basic properties and clinical applications. *Journal of Dentistry*, 35(11), 819–826.

Myshin, H. & Wiens, J. (2005). Factors affecting soft tissue around dental implants: a review of the literature. *Journal of Prosthetic Dentistry*, 94(5), 440–444.

Nevins, M., Kim, D.M., Jum, S.H., Guze, K., Schupbach, P., & Nevins, M. (2010). Histologic evidence of a connective tissue attachment to laser microgrooved abutments: a canine study. *International Journal of Periodontics and Restorative Dentistry*, 30, 245–255.

Page, R. & Schroeder, H.E. (1976). Pathogenesis of inflammatory periodontal disease: a summary of current work. *Laboratory Investigation*, 34, 235–249.

Pecora, G.E., Ceccarelli, R., Bonelli, M., Alexander, H., & Ricci, J.L. (2009). Clinical evaluation of laser microtexturing for soft tissue and bone attachment to dental implants. *Implant Dentistry*, 18(1), 57–66.

Poortinga, A., Bos, R., & Busscher, H. (1999). Measurement of charge transfer during bacterial adhesion to an indium tin oxide surface in a parallel plate flow chamber. *Journal of Microbiological Methods*, 38(3), 183–189.

Prestipino, V. & Ingber, A. (1996). All-ceramic implant abutments: esthetic indications. *Journal of Esthetic and Restorative Dentistry*, 8(1), 255–262.

Quirynen, M., De Soete, M., & Van Steenberghe, D. (2002). Infectious risks for oral implants: a review of the literature. *Clinical Oral Implants Research*, 13(1), 1–19.

Rimondini, L., Cerroni, L., Carrassi, A., & Torricelli, P. (2002). Bacterial colonization of zirconia ceramic surfaces: an in vitro and in vivo study. *International Journal of Oral and Maxillofacial Implants*, 17(6), 793–798.

Rompen, D. (2006). The effect of material charecteristics of surface topography and of implant components and connections on soft tissue integration: a literature review. *Clinical Oral Implants Research*, 17(2), 55–67.

Scarano, A., Piatelli, M., Caputi, S., Favero, G., & Piatelli, A. (2004). Mucosal considerations for osseointegrated implants bacterial adhesion on commercially pure titanium and zirconium oxide disks: an in vivo human study. *Journal of Periodontology*, 75(2), 292–296.

Shapoff, C.A., Lahey, B., Wasserlauf, P., & Kim, D.M. (2010). Radiographic analysis of crestal bone levels around laser-lok collar dental implants. *International Journal of Periodontics and Restorative Dentistry*, 30, 129–137.

Van Brakel, R., Cune, M.S., Van Winkelhoff, A.J., De Putter, C., Verhoeven, J.W., & Van Der Reijden, W. (2010). Early bacterial colonization and soft tissue health around zirconia and titanium abutments: an in vivo study in man. *Clinical Oral Implants Research*, 22(6), 571–577.

Van Brakel, R., Cune, M.S., Van Winkelhoff, A.J., De Putter, C., Verhoeven, J.W., & Van Der Reijden, W. (2011). Early bacterial colonization and soft tissue health around zirconia and titanium abutments: an in vivo study in man. *Clinical Oral Implants Research*, 22(6), 571–577.

Vigolo, P., Fonzi, F., Maizoub, Z., & Cordiolo, G. (2006). An in vitro evaluation of titanium, zirconia, and alumina procera abutments with hexagonal connection. *International Journal of Oral and Maxillofacial Implants*, 21(4), 575–580.

Vigolo, P., Givani, A., Majzoub, Z., & Cordioli, G. (2006). A 4-year prospective study to assess peri-implant hard and soft tissues adjacent to titanium versus gold-alloy abutments in cemented single implant crowns. *Journal of Prosthodontics*, 15(4), 250–256.

Volpe, S., Verrocchi, D., Andersson, P., Gottlow, J., & Sennerby, L. (2008). Comparison of early bacterial colonization of PEEK and titanium healing abutments using real-time PCR. *Applied Osseointegration Research*, 6, 54–56.

Welander, M., Abrahamsson, I., & Berglundh, T. (2008). The mucosal barrier at implant abutments of different materials. *Clinical Oral Implants Research*, 19(7), 635–641.

Wennerberg, A., Sennerby, L., Kultje, C., & Lekholm, U. (2003). Some soft tissue characteristics at implant abutments with different surface topography. A study in humans. *Journal of Clinical Periodontology*, 30(1), 88–94.

Williams, D.F., McNamara, A., Turner, R.M., et al. (1987). Potential of polyetheretherketone (PEEK) and carbon-fibre-reinforced PEEK in medical applications, *Journal of Materials Science Letters*, 6, 188–190.

2
General Information about Implant Abutments

Hamid R. Shafie

Department of Oral and Maxillofacial Surgery, Washington Hospital Center, Washington, DC; and American Institute of Implant Dentistry, Washington, DC

TERMINOLOGY

Dental implant abutments are central to the functional and esthetic aspects of implant treatment. They have a direct impact on the long-term prognosis of this treatment modality. Any abutment can be divided into three segments.

1. *Prosthesis connection segment:* This is the segment of the abutment connected to the prosthesis (Figure 2.1).
2. *Implant connection segment:* this is the segment of the abutment that connects with the implant (Figure 2.2).
3. *Transgingival segment:* This is the segment of the abutment that is surrounded by the gingival tissue above the prosthetic platform of the implant (Figure 2.3).

The implant connection part of the abutment should not be altered, but the other two parts have to be modified in order to optimize the outcome of implant treatment. The prosthesis connection segment should be modified based on the following:

- The size, shape, and emergence profile of the prosthesis.
- The interocclusal or inter-ridge spaces.
- The shape and size of the interdental papilla.

- The desirable embrasure ('V'-shaped gap between the neck of two teeth or crowns that will be filled with gum).
- The clearance required based on the material that will be used to fabricate the final crown. Less reduction is needed for a gold crown and more reduction for PFM (porcelain fused to metal) and all ceramic crowns.

The transgingival part of the abutment needs to be customized based on following:

- The thickness of the gingival above the prosthetic platform of the implant.
- The desirable emergence profile for the tooth that is being replaced.
- The overall prosthetic plan.
- Hygiene and maintenance objectives.

STOCK ABUTMENTS

Stock abutments are generally made of prefabricated titanium. These types of abutments should be modified in the lab or intra-orally so they can support a transitional crown or a final crown or bridge. Implant companies have improved the design of these types of abutments over the years to allow a better emergence profile.

Clinical and Laboratory Manual of Dental Implant Abutments, First Edition. Edited by Hamid R. Shafie.
© 2014 John Wiley & Sons, Inc. Published 2014 by John Wiley & Sons, Inc.

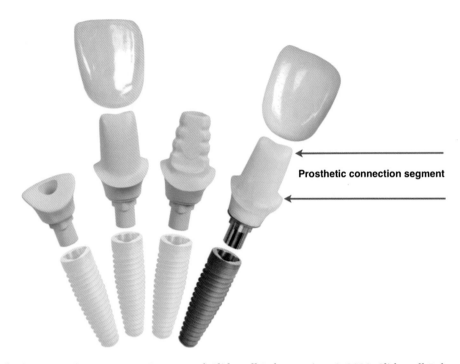

Figure 2.1   Prosthetic connection segment. Courtesy of Glidewell Laboratories. © 2013 Glidewell Laboratories, all rights reserved.

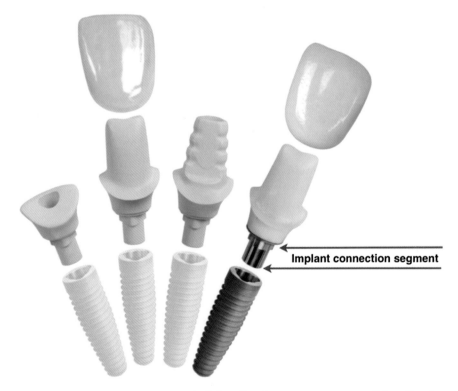

Figure 2.2   Implant connection segment. Courtesy of Glidewell Laboratories. © 2013 Glidewell Laboratories, all rights reserved.

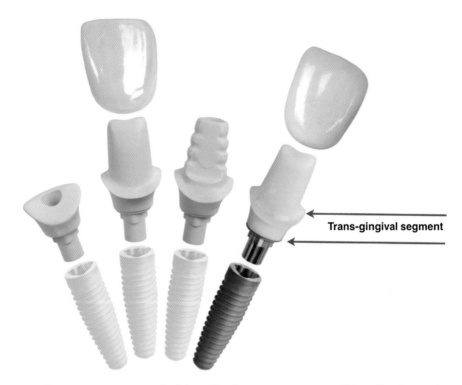

Figure 2.3 Transgingival segment. Courtesy of Glidewell Laboratories. © 2013 Glidewell Laboratories, all rights reserved.

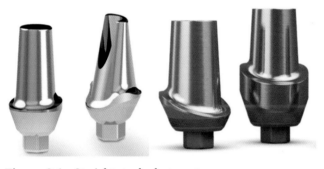

Figure 2.4 Straight stock abutments.

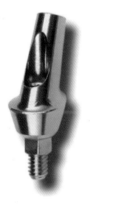

Some clinicians prefer these types of abutments since they are cost effective and allow the dentist to do chairside modifications, making a traditional crown and bride impression instead of an implant-level pick-up impression. However achieving an ideal emergence profile and esthetic with these types of abutments is a challenging task.

The use of stock abutments requires very accurate implant placement in order to minimize reduction of the abutment. A large difference between the trajectory of the implant and that of a desirable crown will require over-reduction of the abutment. In some cases this will compromise the structural integrity of the abutment and may reduce the resistance and retention of the abutment.

The majority of implant manufactures offer straight (Figure 2.4) and angled (Figure 2.5) stock abutments.

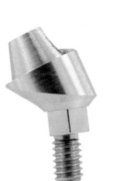

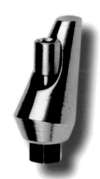

Figure 2.5 Angled stock abutments.

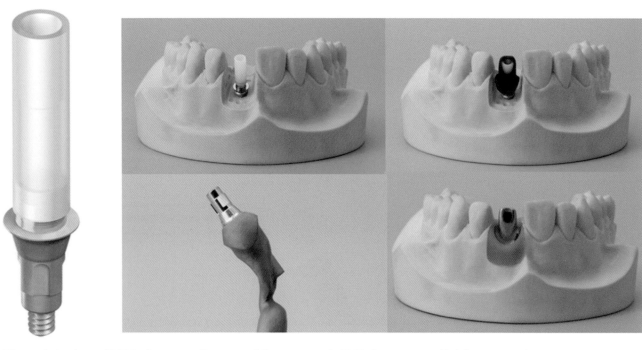

Figure 2.6   A cast UCLA abutment. Courtesy of Straumann. © 2013 Straumann, all rights reserved.

Unfortunately the emergence profile of a crown supported by an angled stock abutment is less than ideal and maintenance will often be difficult for patients.

CUSTOMIZED ABUTMENTS

Customized or custom abutments first became popular after the UCLA abutment was introduced to the market. UCLA abutments provide a means for waxing the emergence profiles of the transgingival portion of the abutment, flexibility in margin level placement, and the correction of angulation problems. Following this success, manufacturers have focused on developing different techniques for fabricating customized abutments (Figure 2.6).

There are three major techniques of customizing implant abutments:

1. *Milling* (starting from a bulky titanium abutment) (Figure 2.7).
2. *Manual modeling* (creating a model for casting or scanning) (Figure 2.8).
3. *Virtual modeling* (designing a model in a virtual environment) (Figure 2.9).

After the fabrication and customization steps, a second process of fine adjustment is required to perfect the abutment fit. The quality and design of the rotary instruments used will have a direct impact on the final outcome of the custom abutment.

CAD/CAM technology has enabled technicians to fabricate patient- or site-specific abutments from tita-

nium and zirconium blanks. The CAD/CAM systems that are used in the fabrication of custom abutments generally consist of three modules:

1. A scanner, which scans a solid model and converts the model into a virtual digital model.
2. Design software, which is used to design the custom abutment.
3. A milling machine, which mills the designed abutment out of titanium or zirconium blanks.

CAD/CAM-fabricated custom abutments have advantages that cannot be matched by cast custom abutments. The titanium and zirconium blanks used by CAD/CAM systems are manufactured using standardized manufacturing procedures under strict quality control. The metals used in the casting process, on the other hand, are subject to many variables, which ultimately make the quality of the final abutment unpredictable.

Custom abutments manufactured from titanium or zirconium blanks are significantly better in quality, strength, and durability compared with cast gold or non-precious custom abutments. This is because during the milling process, titanium and zirconium blanks are not subjected to high casting temperatures that can lead to dimensional discrepancy and eventually to compromised precision of fit.

Note: The same rotary instruments that are used to reshape and modify titanium or zirconium stock abutments are also used during the milling step and post-milling final detailing of the abutment.

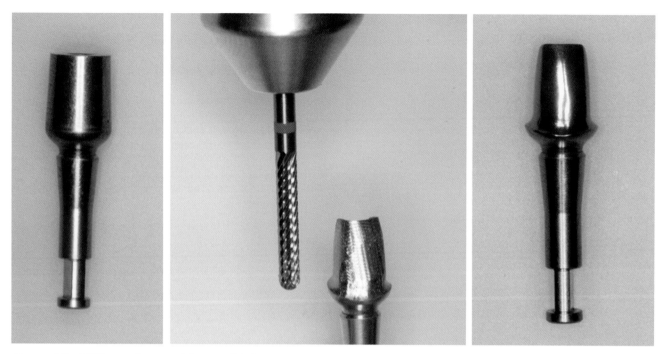

Figure 2.7 Milling and customizing a solid abutment.

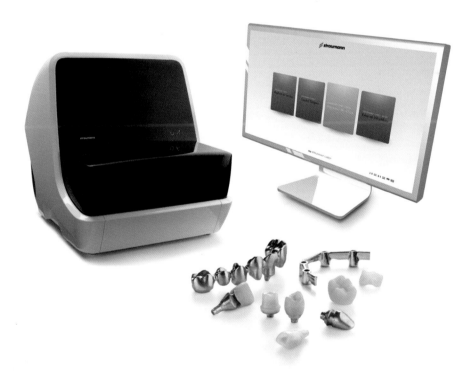

Figure 2.8 Scanning a dental cast that has been fabricated through traditional manual techniques. Courtesy of Straumann. © 2013 Straumann, all rights reserved.

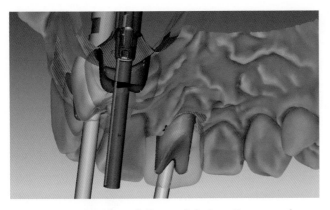

Figure 2.9 Virtual modeling and design. Courtesy of Smart Optics. © 2013 Smart Optics, all rights reserved.

REFERENCES AND ADDITIONAL READING

BioHorizons. Simple Solutions abutment catalogue and prosthetic guide.

Biomet 3i. Restorative manual.

Nobel Biocare. NobelActive procedures and products.

Nobel Biocare. NobelReplace procedures and products.

Straumann. Step by step instructions on prosthetic procedures.

Sybron Implant Solutions. Prosthetic procedures guide.

Zimmer Dental. Step by step instructions on prosthetic procedures.

3

Retaining Abutment Screws

Hamid R. Shafie[1] and Scott Martyna[2]

[1]Department of Oral and Maxillofacial Surgery, Washington Hospital Center, Washington, DC; and American Institute of Implant Dentistry, Washington, DC
[2]Department of Oral and Maxillofacial Surgery, Washington Hospital Center, Washington, DC

INTRODUCTION

The screw that connects the abutment to the implant body is called the prosthetic screw or retaining abutment screw (Figure 3.1). If this small, yet critical, component of the implant system is overlooked, the patient and clinician can face serious challenges. Improper use of the prosthetic screw can have deleterious effects on the implant components, surrounding bone, and final restoration. Prosthetic screws are available in different shapes, sizes, and materials depending on the manufacturer. An understanding of the materials and physical and mechanical aspects are necessary for proper implant–abutment connection, and ultimately implant success. Despite our best efforts, prosthetic failures occasionally occur, and this chapter will also discuss methods for the retrieval of fractured and stripped prosthetic screws.

BASIC TERMINOLOGY

Torque or Moment of Force

This is the tendency of a force to rotate an object about an axis, measured in Newton-centimeters (N-cm). In implant dentistry, this is colloquially referred to as the "tightness" at which the prosthetic screw is secured. Electronic or mechanical torque measuring devices are available to indicate magnitude of torque applied to the prosthetic screw.

Preload or Clamping

In implant dentistry, preload or clamping refers to the linear force, which a stretched prosthetic screw transmits to the abutment and implant body, holding the components together. Preload is measured in Newtons (N). As the prosthetic screw is tightened, the torque applied is transferred to the threads of the prosthetic screw and internal threads of the implant (Figure 3.2). This force clamps the abutment to the implant body. Preload is determined by three factors:

1. Torque, which influences screw head friction, thread friction, and elastic (reversible) deformation of the screw.
2. Screw head geometry.
3. Materials of the screw and abutment, which influence the level of grip (McGlumphy et al. 1998).

Torque has a direct correlation to preload, and is the only factor directly influenced by the clinician. To date no "ideal" preload value has been determined for all prosthetic screws. Because preload is determined by so many different factors, it is recommended to follow each manufacturer's guidelines for each specific screw.

Reverse Torque or Detorque

This is the amount of torque applied *in a counterclockwise direction* to a prosthetic screw to unscrew it from the implant.

Clinical and Laboratory Manual of Dental Implant Abutments, First Edition. Edited by Hamid R. Shafie.
© 2014 John Wiley & Sons, Inc. Published 2014 by John Wiley & Sons, Inc.

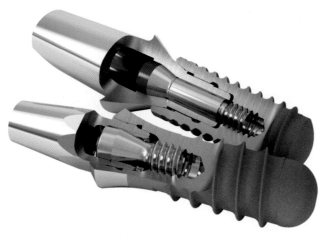

Figure 3.1   Implant, abutment, and retaining screw. Courtesy of Straumann. © Straumann 2013, all rights reserved.

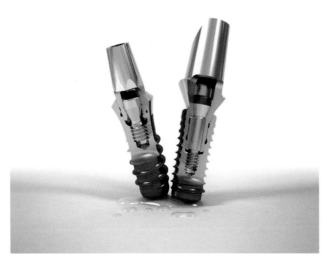

Figure 3.2   Retaining prosthetic screw. Courtesy of Thommen Medical. © Thommen Medical 2013, all rights reserved.

Screw Loosening

This refers to the unwanted rotation of the prosthetic screw in a counterclockwise direction. Screw loosening is one of the most common complications encountered in implant dentistry (Ekfeldt et al. 1994). Loose screws are at a significantly higher risk of screw fracture. Binon and McHugh (1996) suggest multiple reasons for screw loosening:

* Poor tightening.
* An inadequate prosthesis.
* Poor component fit.
* Excessive loading.
* Settling of the screw.
* Elasticity of the bone.

Settling or Torque Loss

This is a decrease in preload as a result of burnishing of both the internal implant threads and the prosthetic screw threads. Unlike screw loosening, the prosthetic screw does not "unscrew." The frictional forces between the components are decreased as a result of creep and stress relaxation, which eventually will cause a decrease in preload. This is a normal occurrence which should be anticipated and corrected by retorqueing the prosthetic screw to the recommended moment force after a period of time. It is recommended that the prosthetic screws be retorqued 10 minutes after initial placement and periodically thereafter (Winkler et al. 2003; Cantwell and Hobkirk 2004). Torque loss will also occur over longer periods of time. It is recommended to retorque the prosthetic screw at each recall visit. This has not been shown to have any harmful effects on the implant joint stability (Delben et al. 2011).

ABUTMENT SCREW MECHANICS

Prosthetic screws are manufactured in a variety of different shapes, sizes, and materials (Figure 3.3). It is important to understand the implication of this aspect on the final prosthetic outcome. Although a seemingly small and simple piece, the mechanics of the prosthetic screw are fairly complex. Literally, this piece holds the implant system together and thus it requires sophisticated engineering to provide the best possible prosthetic results.

Shape and Size

Like any other screw, there are three basic components of the prosthetic retaining screw (Figure 3.4):

1. *Screw head:* The head contains the driver fitting site, which is used to rotate the screw into position. Various driver fitting site types are available, including slot (flat-head), Phillips, Robertson (square), hex, and star. By far, the most common type used in implant dentistry is the hex type. It is critically important to use the appropriate corresponding driver to prevent screw head stripping.
2. *Shank:* The shank is the unthreaded portion of the screw below the head. It is variable in length depending on the geometry of the components that are being held together.
3. *Thread:* Without going into too much complexity, the thread can come in a myriad of different dimensions. This portion of the screw engages the internal threads of the implant and provides the surfaces onto which force is transmitted and converted to preload. The internal threads of the implant and

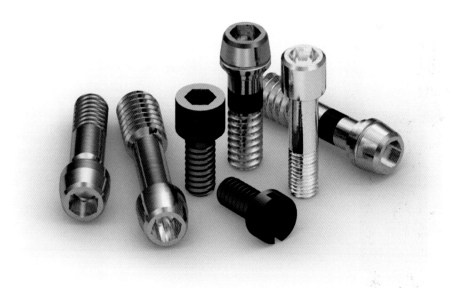

Figure 3.3 Various retaining prosthetic screws. Courtesy of Dentsply. © 2013 Dentsply, all rights reserved.

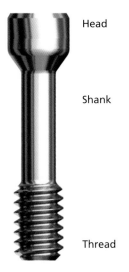

Head

Shank

Thread

Figure 3.4 Parts of the retaining prosthetic screw. Courtesy of Maxillent. © 2013 Maxillent, all rights reserved.

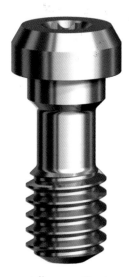

Figure 3.5 Commercially pure titanium screw. Courtesy of Nobel Biocare. © Nobel Biocare 2013, all rights reserved.

those of the prosthetic retaining screw must be 100% compatible.

ABUTMENT SCREW MATERIALS

Motosch (1976) studied the basic mechanics of screws and noted that only 10% of the initial rotational torque forces are transferred to preload, the rest being used to overcome the friction of the threads sliding past one another. Materials science has focused on decreasing the amount of friction to allow greater preload values for the amount of toque applied.

Commercially Pure Titanium

This is one of the most common materials used to manufacture prosthetic screws (Figure 3.5). This material generates the least amount of preload for a given torque when compared with other materials. After applying desirable torque, commercially pure titanium prosthetic screws only undergo elastic (reversible) deformation, and can thus be used multiple times. These screws are appropriate for use with temporary restorations and laboratory procedures. They are not recommended for use with final restorations.

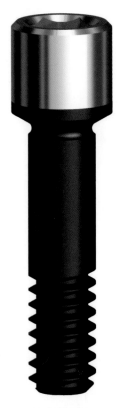

Figure 3.6 Carbon-coated titanium screw. Courtesy of Nobel Biocare. © Nobel Biocare 2013, all rights reserved.

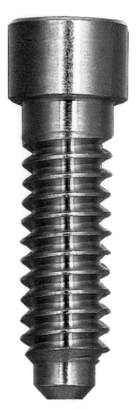

Figure 3.7 Gold-plated screw. Courtesy of Biomet 3i. © Biomet 3i 2013, all rights reserved.

Coated or Treated Titanium

In an effort to decrease friction and increase preload, manufacturers began coating and treating titanium screws (Figure 3.6). Coatings and treatments can include gold, tungsten carbon carbide, and nitrides. Titanium treated in such a way to include different chemicals is called titanium alloy. These alloys are expensive to manufacture, but have very high tensile strength and toughness. In general, coated and treated prosthetic screws are able to provide higher preload than non-pure titanium prosthetic screws, and are more capable of maintaining preload after cyclical loading.

Gold

Gold prosthetic screws are available in pure gold and in gold alloys that contain other elements to strengthen the metal (Figure 3.7). Gold can act as a dry lubricant, decreasing the amount of friction between the threads as the screw is tightened. This allows increased rotation and elongation of the screw for a given torque, and thus a greater preload. These screws are least likely to loosen over time. However, gold screws, especially those of high carat, are subject to plastic (irreversible) deformation, and thus are only indicated for single use. It is recommended that before final delivery of the abutment and prosthesis, the clinician use titanium screws and to only use gold screws during final delivery.

Implant manufacturers are now making implant components that are ostensibly interchangeable between systems. However, even the slightest incompatibility in physical characteristics and chemical composition of implant components affects preload and can have an effect on settling and screw loosening (Kim et al. 2012). Despite a seemingly accurate fit, slight differences in thread pitch or materials incompatibility can have significant long-term consequences and ultimately result in failure. Thus, it is always recommended using the same company for implant, abutment, screw driver, and prosthetic screw. Table 3.1 lists the screw materials that are currently available from major implant companies.

SPECIAL CONSIDERATIONS

Implant Connection Types

When deciding on an implant, it is also important to consider how different connection types relation to

Table 3.1 Prosthetic screws available from the major implant companies

Implant company	Commercially pure titanium	Treated or coated titanium	Gold
BioHorizons			
Zimmer		✔	
Nobel	✔	✔	
Astra	✔		
Straumann		✔	
Biomet 3i		✔	✔ *

*Surgical grade stainless steel with gold plating.

the prosthetic retaining screw. Internal connection implants have been shown to have significantly better torque maintenance when compared with external hex implants (Park et al. 2010; Jorge et al. 2013). When considering different types of internal connections, it has been shown that the prosthetic retaining screw torque can have a significant impact on the vertical height of the final restoration in those implants with Morse taper connections (Yilmaz et al. 2013). For this reason, it is advised that the laboratory technician torques the retaining screw to the full amount during laboratory procedures to accurately simulate the vertical position of the final prosthesis.

Single versus Multi-unit Implant Restorations

Jemt (1991) has demonstrated that screw loosening occurs most commonly on single crown implant restorations. During recall examinations it is recommended that screw-retained restorations are periodically retorqued, especially with single-unit restorations.

Achieving Optimal Torque

Always follow the manufacturer's recommendations for the amount of torque to apply to the prosthetic screw. Too little toque will result in inadequate preload and screw loosening, and too much can also, paradoxically, lead to screw loosening. It has been demonstrated that when preload values over 60–75% of the elastic (reversible) limit of the prosthetic screw material are achieved there is actually some amount of plastic (irreversible) change that occurs, which ultimately results in screw loosening (Haack et al. 1995). Griffith (1987) suggested that the optimal preload for a given screw is 75% of the force required to exceed its ultimate breaking strength. Excessive values of preload can also transmit stresses on the implant collar and marginal bone, leading to crestal bone loss

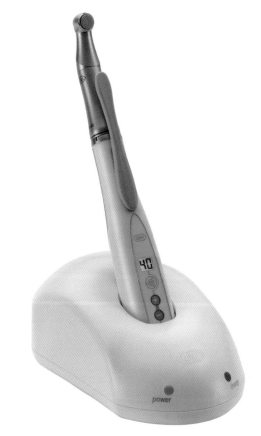

Figure 3.8 Electronic torque driver. Courtesy of W&H Group. © W&H Group 2013, all rights reserved.

(Khraisat 2012). For the most accurate measurement of torque value it is recommended to use a torque-limiting device.

Torque-limiting Devices

There are four common torque-limiting devices used in implant dentistry:[nl]

1. Electronic torque drivers (Figure 3.8).
2. Toggle-type devices (Figure 3.9).
3. Beam-type wrenches (Figure 3.10).
4. Finger torqueing.

A study by Hill and colleagues (2007) demonstrated that maximal finger tightening varied between 4.0 and 21.7 N-cm, with very few of the study participants being able to reach torque values above 20 N-cm. Electronic torque drivers have been shown to be the most accurate, with toggle-type devices having the most variability apart from finger tightening (McCracken et al. 2010).

Screw Drivers

Screw drivers come in various shapes and sizes that correspond to the head of the prosthetic screw.

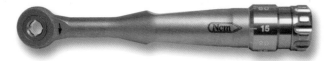

Figure 3.9 Toggle-type wrench. Courtesy of Osseous Technologies of America. © Osseous Technologies of America 2013, all rights reserved.

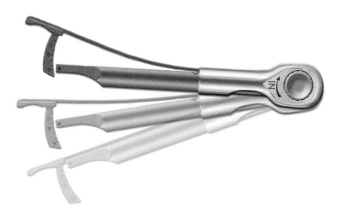

Figure 3.10 Beam-type wrench. Courtesy of Biomet 3i. © Biomet 3i 2013, all rights reserved.

Common types of drivers include slot (flat-head), Robertson (square), hex, and torx (Figure 3.11, Table 3.2). Drivers come with shafts of various length and can be connected to a wrench or electronic driver (as shown in Figure 3.8), or be a simple thumb driver (Figure 3.12). Table 3.3 lists some of the common drivers used by the major implant companies.

ABUTMENT SCREW FAILURE

Screw Fracture

Fracture of the prosthetic screw was once considered a fairly common complication in implant dentistry (Figure 3.13) (Goodacre et al. 1999, 2003). Kreissl and colleagues (2007) found the incidence of screw fracture over a 5-year period to be as high as 3.9%. The most commonly cited reasons for prosthetic screw fracture are inadequate or excessive preload, screw loosening, and unfavorable forces on the implant components (Eckert et al. 2000; Taylor et al. 2000; Bakaeen et al. 2001). Ultimately the reason for screw fracture is a material failure. Oftentimes the screw will fracture prior to any irreversible damage to the implant or prosthesis, thus acting as a fail-safe. Should this situation arise, it is critical to assess and correct the most likely reason for failure to prevent future screw loosening or fracture.

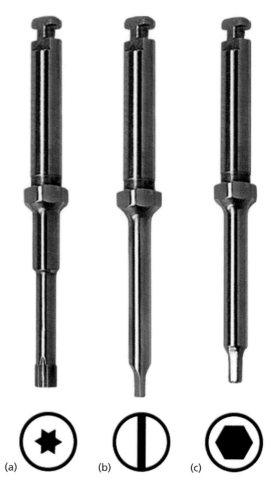

(a)   (b)   (c)

Figure 3.11 (a) Torx, (b) slot, and (c) hex drivers. Yilmaz and McGlumphy (2011).

Multiple reports in the literature have offered techniques to salvage or remove the fractured screws (Walia et al. 2012; Francis et al. 2013; Yilmaz and McGlumphy 2013). Screw-retrieval kits are available from various dental implant companies. However, most of these systems use aggressive motorized devices that increase the risk of damage to the implant, which would result in an unrestorable implant.

The following algorithm is proposed when dealing with fractured prosthetic screws (Figure 3.14). The first step is removing the coronal portion of the fractured screw and obtain visual access, with ample light to see the remaining screw fragment. Sometimes if the fracture is coronal enough, removal with an explorer and hemostat is possible. Failing this, use an ultrasonic scaler with a blunt tip. Try to vibrate the fractured screw fragment and assess if it is loose within the internal implant threads. If the fractured piece is loose, retrieval should be attempted. If it is not loose, assess the level of the screw fracture line and determine if removal of the fractured piece is absolutely necessary to utilize the implant. If there are enough free internal implant threads above the fractured part of the screw,

Table 3.2 Different types of implant screw drivers and their tips

Specifications	Latch type screwdriver	Tips	Specifications	Latch type screwdriver	Tips	Specifications	Latch type screwdriver	Tips
21 mm IMPLANT SCREW DRIVER #1, TORX T6		✦	26.5 mm IMPLANT SCREW DRIVER #4, ALLEN KEY, 0.3MM SIDES		⬡	21 mm IMPLANT SCREW DRIVER #8, ALLEN KEY, 1.2MM SIDES		⬡
26.5 mm IMPLANT SCREW DRIVER #1, TORX T7		✦	21.mm IMPLANT SCREW DRIVER #5, ALLEN KEY, 0.5MM SIDES		⬡	26.5 mm IMPLANT SCREW DRIVER #8, ALLEN KEY, 1.2MM SIDES		⬡
21 mm IMPLANT SCREW DRIVER #2, FLAT, 1.6MM WIDE		⊖	26.5 mm IMPLANT SCREW DRIVER #5, ALLEN KEY, 0.5MM SIDES		⬡	21 mm IMPLANT SCREW DRIVER #9, ALLEN KEY, 1.8MM SIDES		⬡
26.5 mm IMPLANT SCREW DRIVER #2, FLAT, 1.6AAM WIDE		⊖	21 mm IMPLANT SCREW DRIVER #6, ALLEN KEY, 0.9MM SIDES		⬡	26.5 mm IMPLANT SCREW DRIVER #9, ALLEN KEY, 1.8MM SIDES		⬡
21 mm IMPLANT SCREW DRIVER #3, FLAT, 2.0MM WIDE		⊖	26.5 mm IMPLANT SCREW DRIVER #6, ALLEN KEY, 0.9MM SIDES		⬡	IMPLANT SCREWDRIVER SET		
26.5 mm IMPLANT SCREW DRIVER #3, FLAT, 2.0MM WIDE		⊖	21 mm IMPLANT SCREW DRIVER #7, ALLEN KEY, 1.0MM SIDES		⬡			
21 mm IMPLANT SCREW DRIVER #4, ALLEN KEY, 0.3MM SIDES		⬡	26.5 mm IMPLANT SCREW DRIVER #7, ALLEN KEY, 1.0MM SIDES		⬡			

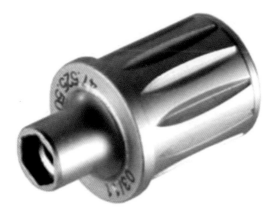

Figure 3.12 Thumb driver. Maalhagh-Fard and Jacobs (2010).

Table 3.3 Drivers produced by the major implant companies

Driver	Company
Hex 0.035	Ankylos, Biohorizons, Biomet 3i
Hex 0.048	Biomet 3i, Nobel Biocare
Hex 0.050	Astra, BioHorizons, Zimmer
Square 0.050	Nobel Biocare
Torx	Replace Select, Straumann

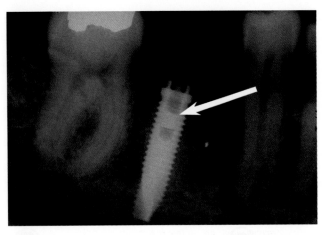

Figure 3.13   Fractured screw. Yilmaz and McGlumphy (2011).

continue the restorative steps by utilizing a shorter retaining screw. Use a perio probe to measure how much length of a new prosthetic retaining screw should be removed. Using the titanium adjustment kit (Vitality Kit 1826, Jota), shorten the new screw to the desired length. When attaching the prosthetic abutment, ensure that you are able to torque the retaining screw to the necessary preload. If you are unable to reach the recommended preload, the retained screw fragment will need to be removed.

To attempt removal of the retained screw fragment, start by placing a small dimple in the center of the screw fragment with an ultrasonic instrument using a fine tip. Extend the dimple to the periphery of the screw on either side to crease a flat-head drive on the surface of the screw fragment. Be careful not to damage

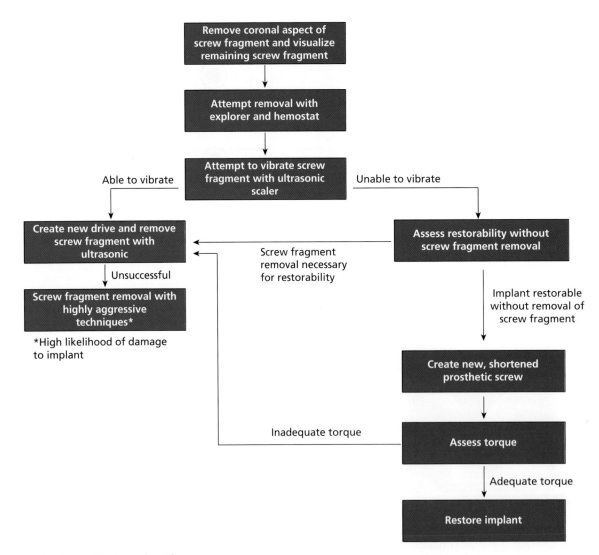

Figure 3.14   Screw fracture algorithm.

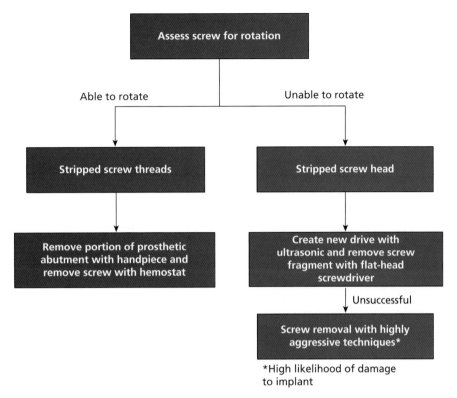

Figure 3.15 Stripped screw algorithm.

the internal implant threads at the periphery of the screw. Use a flat-head screw driver to engage the created groove and attempt to rotate the screw fragment in a counterclockwise direction.

Note: If the internal implant threads are damaged during the fractured screw removal that implant will become useless and restorable. Ultimately the implant should be removed.

Screw Stripping

This can refer to stripping of the head of the screw, or stripping of the threads of the screw. This situation most often results when excessive forces are placed on the screw, or when an ill-fitting or incompatible driver is used. It is advised that only the correct driver from the same manufacturer is used when placing prosthetic screws. Many of the same techniques for the retrieval of fractured screws can also be used for stripped screws. An algorithm is proposed here for the retrieval of stripped screws (Figure 3.15).

Assess if the screw is able to be rotated with the correct driver. If the correct driver can engage the screw head, but rotation of the driver does not back the screw out, you have to assume that the screw threads are stripped. In this situation, removal of a portion of the surrounding prosthetic abutment may be required to have a physical grasp on the screw for removal (Figure 3.16) (Maalhagh-Fard and Jacobs

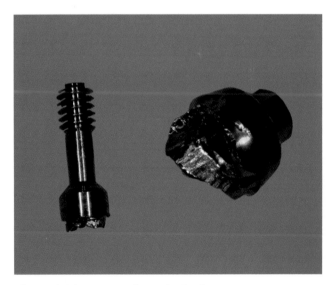

Figure 3.16 Damaged prosthetic abutment.

2010). Be careful not to damage the implant during this process. When sufficient access is available around the retaining screw, use a hemostat to lift the screw out of the implant.

If the correct driver is unable to engage the screw head, the technique described above is used to create a new drive in the head of the implant. A flat-head screw driver can then be used to remove the prosthetic screw. In all situations, careful assessment of the internal aspect of the implant under magnification is recommended to identify possible damage to the internal threads of the implant.

REFERENCES AND ADDITIONAL READING

Bakaeen, L.G., Winkler, S., & Neff, P.A. (2001). The effect of implant diameter, restoration design, and occlusal table variations on screw loosening of posterior single-tooth implant restorations. *Journal of Oral Implantology*, 27, 63-72.

Binon, P.P. & McHugh, M.J. (1996). The effect of eliminating implant/abutment rotational misfit on screw joint stability. *International Journal of Prosthodontics*, 9, 511–519.

Cantwell, A. & Hobkirk, J.A. (2004). Preload loss in gold prosthesis-retaining prosthetic screws as a function of time. *International Journal of Oral and Maxillofacial Implants*, 19, 124–132.

Delben, J.A., Gomes, E.A., Barao, V.A.R., & Assuncao, W.G. (2011). Evaluation of the effect of retightening and mechanical cycling on preload maintenance on retention screws. *International Journal of Oral and Maxillofacial Implants*, 26(2), 251–255.

Eckert, S.E., Meraw, S.J., Cal, E., & Ow, R.K. (2000). Analysis of incidence and associated factors with fractured implants: a retrospective study. *International Journal of Oral and Maxillofacial Implants*, 15, 662–667.

Ekfeldt, A., Carlsson, G.E., & Borjesson, G. (1994). Clinical evaluation of single-tooth restorations supported by osseointegrated implants: a retrospective study. *International Journal of Oral and Maxillofacial Implants*, 9, 179–183.

Francis, L., Zeenath, H., Lylajam, S., & Harshakumar, K. (2013). Implant screw fracture. *Journal of Dental Implants*, 3(2), 181.

Goodacre, C.J., Bernai, G., Rungcharassaeng, K., & Kan, J.Y. (2003). Clinical complications with implants and impiant prostheses. *Journal of Prosthetic Dentistry*, 90, 121–132.

Goodacre, C.J., Kan, J.Y., & Rungcharassaeng, K. (1999). Clinical complications of osseointegrated implants. *Journal of Prosthetic Dentistry*, 81, 537–552.

Griffith, H.T. (1987). Suggested tightening torques for structural bolts. In *Torque Tensioning: A Ten Part Compilation*. Stow, OH: Fastener Technology.

Haack, J.E., Sakaguchi, R.L., Sun, T., & Coffey, J.P. (1995). Elongation and preload stress in dental implant retaining prosthetic screws. *International Journal of Oral and Maxillofacial Implants*, 10, 529–536.

Hill, E.E., Phillips, S.M., & Breeding, L.C. (2007). Implant abutment screw torque generated by general dentists using a hand driver in a limited access space simulating the mouth. *Journal of Oral Implantology*, 33(5), 277–279.

Jemt, T. (1991). Consecutively inserted fixed prostheses supported by Branemark implants in edentulous jaws: a study of treatment from the time of prosthesis placement to the first annual checkup. *International Journal of Oral and Maxillofacial Implants*, 6, 270–276.

Jorge, J.R.P., Barao, V.A.R., Delben, J.A., & Assuncao, W.G. (2013). The role of implant/abutment system on torque maintenance of retention screws and vertical misfit of implant-supported crowns before and after mechanical cycling. *International Journal of Oral and Maxillofacial Implants*, 28(2), 415–422.

Khraisat, A. (2012). Influence of abutment screw preload on stress distribution in marginal bone. *International Journal of Oral and Maxillofacial Implants*, 27(2), 303–307.

Kim, S.K., Koak, J.Y., Heo, S.J., Taylor, T.D., Ryoo, S., & Lee, S.Y. (2012). Screw loosening with interchangeable abutments in internally connected implants after cyclic loading. *International Journal of Oral and Maxillofacial Implants*, 27(1), 42–47.

Kreissl, M.E., Gerds, T., Muche, R., Heydecke, G., & Strub, J.R. (2007). Technical complications of implant-supported fixed partial dentures in partially edentulous cases after an average observation period of 5 years. *Clinical Oral Implants Research*, 18, 720–6.

Maalhagh-Fard, A. & Jacobs, L.C. (2010). Retrieval of a stripped retaining prosthetic screw: a clinical report. *Journal of Prosthetic Dentistry*, 104(4), 212–215.

McCracken, M.S., Mitchell, L., Hegde, R., & Mavalli, M.D. (2010). Variability of mechanical torque-limiting devices in clinical service at a US dental school. *Journal of Prosthodontics*, 19(1), 20–24.

McGlumphy, E.A., Mendel, D.A., & Holloway, J.A. (1998). Implant screw mechanics. *Dent Clinics of North America*, 42, 71–89.

Motosch, N. (1976). Development of design charts for bolts preloaded up to the plastic range. *Journal of Engineering for Industry*, 98, 849–851.

Park, J.-K., Choi, J.-U., Jeon, Y.-C., Choi, K.-S., & Jeong, C.-M. (2010). Effects of retaining prosthetic screw coating on implant preload. *Journal of Prosthodontics*, 19(6), 458–464.

Taylor, T.D., Agar, J.R., & Vogiatzi, T. (2000). Implant prosthodontics: current perspective and future directions. *International Journal of Oral and Maxillofacial Implants*, 15, 66–75.

Walia, M., Arora, S., Luthra, R., & Walia, P.K. (2012). Removal of fractured dental implant screw using a new technique: a case report. *Journal of Oral Implantology*, 38(6), 747–750.

Winkler, S., Ring, K., Ring, J.D., & Boberick, K.G. (2003). Implant screw mechanics and the settling effect: an overview. *Journal of Oral Implantology*, 29(5), 242–245.

Yilmaz, B. & McGlumphy, E.A. (2011). A technique to retrieve fractured implant screws. *Journal of Prosthetic Dentistry*, 105(2), 137–138.

Yilmaz, B. & McGlumphy, E.A. (2013). A technique to salvage a single implant-supported dental prosthesis having a nonretrievable implant screw fragment. *Journal of Oral Implantology*, 39(1), 81–83.

Yilmaz, B., Seidt, J.D., McGlumphy, E.A., & Clelland, N.L. (2013). Displacement of screw-retained single crowns into implants with conical internal connections. *International Journal of Oral and Maxillofacial Implants*, 28(3), 803–806.

4

Different Implant–Abutment Connections

Hamid R. Shafie[1] and Bryan A. White[2]

[1]Department of Oral and Maxillofacial Surgery, Washington Hospital Center, Washington, DC; and American Institute of Implant Dentistry, Washington, DC
[2]Private Practice, Gilbert, AZ

INTRODUCTION

The history of abutment connections began with Branemark's landmark discovery of the dental implant. Branemark's original implant was composed of a 0.7 mm external hex with a butt joint. Initially there was little interest in antirotational features of the abutment connection because implants were used to treat fully edentulous patients and were connected together with a one-piece metal substructure. The external hex portion of the implant was added to the design to enable surgical placement of the implant.

Times changed and clinicians started using implants for the replacement of single teeth. This new application meant that abutment connections were subjected to an increased level of forces. This challenge has encouraged research and the development of better forms of abutment connections within the implant dentistry.

CHRONOLOGICAL DEVELOPMENT OF ABUTMENT CONNECTIONS

The abutment modifications that have occurred are vast and complex. For example, the external hex underwent several modifications of height and width. Besides altering the size, other modifications were also made in an effort to improve upon the original external hex design.

A major paradigm shift came with the evolution of the internal connection. Each implant company has developed their own design of the internal connection, resulting in a confusing variation in terminology and types of connections.

Terminology

- *External connection:* A connection feature that extends superior to the coronal portion of the implant. **Note**: Although the external hex connection is the most common there are other types (i.e. external spline or external octagon)
- *Internal connection:* A connection feature that extends inferior to the coronal portion of the implant and is located inside the implant body
- *Hexagonal:* A six-sided shape used at the abutment–implant interface as an antirotational feature
- *External hexagon or external "hex":* An external connection that is used as an antirotational and indexing feature
- *Internal hexagon or internal "hex":* An internal connection that is used as an antirotational and indexing feature

The initial relationship between the abutment and implant body was mainly associated with external connections. Over time the simple butt joint has

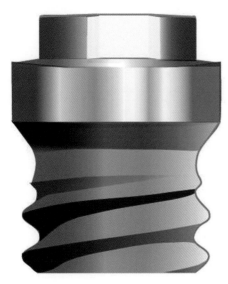

Figure 4.1 External hex.

evolved into slip-fit and friction-fit joints. The internal connections have splintered into a multitude of options from octagonal, hexagonal, cone screw, cylinder hex, spline, tri-channel to cam tube – to name just a few.

This chapter examines the basic differences between the abutment connections on the market and should enable readers to make educated decisions in selecting implant–abutment connections.

EXTERNAL HEX CONNECTIONS

There are a number of advantages and disadvantages of the external hex connection (Figure 4.1) shown in the boxes.

Advantages of the external hex connection

- Long-term follow-up data are available
- Compatibility among multiple implant systems
- Solutions to complications are found throughout the literature due to their extensive use

Disadvantages of the external hex connection

- Higher prevalence of screw loosening
- Higher prevalence of rotational misfit
- Less esthetic results
- Inadequate microbial seal

Prosthetic success remains high with the external connection but the most common prosthetic complication is screw loosening when implants are used to replace a missing single tooth. Multiple studies have

shown screw loosening to be anywhere from 6% to 48% with external connection devices.

Screw loosening can create serious challenges for the clinician and patient and diminishes a practitioner's chairside time, which is the most valuable asset a practitioner has. In addition, screw loosening can be frustrating for patients, which damages the patient's trust in the clinician's qualifications and abilities.

When an external hex implant is used to replace a single tooth, the weakest link between the implant, abutment connection, screw, and bone is the screw. This is because with this connection type the screw alone secures the abutment.

External Connection

The initial 0.7 mm external connection, being short in length, provided only limited screw engagement. The original narrow platform associated with the external hex connection created a short fulcrum arm, which also increased screw loosening due to adverse tipping forces. Consequently, the short and narrow external connections made screw loosening a common occurrence. Research clearly indicates that screw loosening is more common with external connections. The seriousness of screw loosening resulted in manufacturers implementing major modifications to the external hex connection.

Modifications

The first solution to overcome the adverse force distribution and instability of the abutment connection was increasing the width and height of the external hex connection. Currently available external hex heights range from 0.7 to 1.2 mm and widths from 2.0 to 3.4 mm, depending on the manufacturer. These adjustments increased the fulcrum arm and deepened the abutment screw engagement, thus limiting the tipping forces on abutment screws and reducing the prevalence of screw loosening.

Retaining Prosthetic Screw

Another aspect that was modified to lessen screw loosening was the design of the retaining prosthetic screw itself. As a screw is tightened with torque it elongates and produces tension between the abutment and implant. Elastic recovery then occurs within the screw, which creates a "clamping force" binding the abutment and the implant.

Preload is defined as the difference between screw elongation and elastic recovery. This determines the "clamping force" which binds the abutment and implant together. Screw loosening occurs when the forces acting on the implant are greater than the "clamping force" or preload of the screw.

Modifications

Several modifications have been made to improve upon the design of Branemark's original abutment screw. In 2000, Binon noted screw modifications that included the shank, number of threads, diameter, length, thread design, and torque applications of the abutment screw.

Other changes have focused on the material of the screw itself. Haack et al. (1995) suggested that gold screws were superior to titanium. Haack noted that, at manufacturers' torque recommendations, the mean preload using a gold screw was greater than that of titanium. Reports have shown gold alloy screws to achieve over twice the preloads of titanium alloy screws. A greater preload minimizes screw loosening.

Rotational Misfit and Screw Loosening

Rotational misfit is the misfit between the implant and the abutment. This rotational freedom of the abutment itself on the implant contributes to screw loosening and may lead to micro-movements during loading. In addition, when components do not seat properly, tightening a screw may damage the threads within the implant or on the screw itself. Either way the misfit of the abutment and implant leads to screw loosening.

Studies have shown that a rotational misfit of less than 2 degrees provides a stable screw joint, thus limiting screw loosening. However, the rotational misfit of the external hex connection was originally shown to be between 3 and 10 degrees, providing a further cause of screw loosening.

Modifications

Once taller and wider external hex connections were introduced, the problem of rotational misfit improved. From a manufacturing standpoint, machining a larger hex is much easier and results in enhanced precision of fit and a reduction in rotational misfit.

In addition, other designs were developed to eliminate the degree of rotational misfit. For example, 1.5 degrees of taper among hex flats was introduced, which creates a friction fit between the abutment and implant. Another design involved adding micro-stops in the corners of the abutment hexagon that engages the implant hexagon. Both these designs aimed to limit the misfit, which in turn limits micro-movements and screw loosening.

INTERNAL CONNECTIONS

External connection modifications have reduced the problem of screw loosening. However, overcoming the esthetic and microbial seal issues warranted a novel approach to the design of the abutment connection. Rather than modify the existing abutment, a new concept was developed – that of the internal connection. This shift revolutionized the market. Now numerous variations of internal connections are available from the different implant manufacturers.

Advantages of the internal connection

- Less screw loosening
- Better esthetics
- Improved microbial seal
- Better joint strength
- More platform switching options

Disadvantages of the internal connection

- The weakest link is the bone rather than the retaining prosthetic screw
- There is less historical literature on internal connections than external connections

---

Force Distributions

With an internal connection the weakest link between the implant, abutment connection, screw, and bone is the bone. The force distribution with an internal connection loads deep within the implant wall and distributes out towards the bone. This force distribution shields the forces placed on the screw itself, thus dramatically reducing screw loosening. Levine et al.'s study in 1999 showed screw loosening with conical internal abutment connections to be as low as 3.5%. This was a remarkable improvement from the external connection record, where studies found levels of screw loosening ranging from 6% to 48%.

However, some practitioners do not consider the load transfer feature of the internal connection to be a positive improvement. They argue that if an implant–abutment connection receives excessive forces due to traumatic occlusion or implant malpositioning, screw loosing is easier to deal with than crestal bone loss around the implant.

Rotational Misfit and Screw Loosening

The rotational misfit found in internal connection designs is significantly less than that of the original external hex connection. Some internal connections have essentially eliminated rotational misfit by using a friction-fit design. The precise fit between implant and abutment limits any micro-motion between them, thus limiting screw loosening.

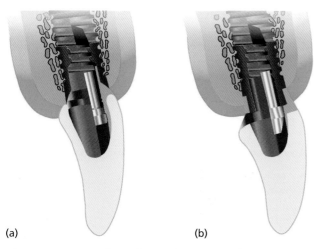

(a)   (b)

Figure 4.2 Note the esthetic advantage with an internal connection (a) over that of an external connection (b). Courtesy of Zimmer Dental. © 2012 Zimmer Dental, all rights reserved.

Esthetics

With esthetic zone restorations, the buccal aspect of the prosthesis needs to have enough bulk of ceramic to achieve an ideal color and esthetic outcome. In addition, an esthetically pleasing restoration requires a coronal transition depth from the implant–abutment connection to the gingival margin. This maintains a proper emergence profile and masks the unesthetic metal connection.

External connections are limited in their ability to provide the necessary transition depth or bulk required for esthetic restorations. They may also occasionally appear bulky with an unesthetic emergence profile. Also, external connections may have metal exposed at the finish line level since an expansive abutment cuff height is required to house the external connection of the implant.

Internal connections (Figure 4.2) are undeniably superior in their ability to provide an esthetic restoration. They permit a sufficient bulk of restoration while at the same time permitting a smooth buccal contour. In addition, the internal connection may provide a better prosthetic emergence profile because technicians can trim the abutment accurately.

Microbial Seal

Any implantologist has experienced a foul odor when an implant abutment is removed. This is due to a leakage of saliva and bacteria into the micro-gap between the implant and abutment, providing a space for micro-organisms to accumulate and thrive. This collection not only creates toxins that cause the unpleasant odor when the abutment is removed, but also increases inflammation at the implant–abutment junction that will eventually cause crestal bone loss.

Internal connections have a greater potential for obtaining a microbial seal between the abutment and implant than do external connections. This microbial seal is achieved due to the precise fit between the abutment and implant, excluding even the smallest microbes. This is a major advantage, although some internal connections fare better than others in this respect.

Many implant companies have capitalized on their superior microbial seal to market their implant systems. For example, Bicon's study in 2004 verified that their internal morse taper connection provides a hermetic seal that does not permit bacteria to leak from outside-in or from inside-out the abutment connection (Dibart et al. 2005). Mairgünther and Netwig in 1992 showed that the Ankylos abutment connection could provide a vacuum seal for 60 hours.

Most internal connection designs have entered the market with studies promoting their ability to provide a microbial seal.

Superior Joint Strength

Mollersten et al., back in 1997, concluded that deep joints were more likely to resist bending forces than shallow joints. The shallow 0.7 mm external hex connections are simply outdated as deep internal joint connections have greater joint strength. This superior joint strength is particularly important under increased load-bearing areas like the molar regions.

Some practitioners argue that the main reason to use internal connections is because they are esthetically superior in the anterior area. Others maintain that their main attraction is due to their superior joint strength in the posterior area. And some still argue that they prefer internal connections because they are less of a hassle with little screw loosening. Regardless of where implants are placed in the mouth, most clinicians now consider internal connections to be preferable to external connections. It is no surprise that there is such a wide variety of internal connections on the market today for clinicians to choose from.

Platform Switching

Platform switching is a method of preventing crestal bone loss. Although this feature is offered by internal and external connections, the internal connection design uses platform switching more often. To platform switch, the diameter of the abutment is narrower than that of the implant. For example, a 5 mm diameter implant might be used with a 4 mm diameter abutment. Traditionally, the diameter of the implant and the abutment were identical.

Table 4.1 Friction-fit connections on the market

Company	Connection	Unique features
Zimmer: Screw-Vent	Internal hexagon	1.5 mm deep internal connection
BioHorizonss: Tapered Internal	Internal hexagon	Spiralock screw technology
Biomet 3i: Osseotite Certain	Hexagonal and dodecagaonal antirotational features	Audible "click" when seated *Platform switching*
Bicon	Morse taper	No abutment retaining screw necessary. Inherent *platform switching*
Straumann: synOcta	Cone screw	Internal octagonal antirotational feature Inherent *platform switching*
Astra Tech: Astra	Cone screw	Dodecagonal antirotational feature Inherent *platform switching*
Ankylos	Cone screw	No additional antirotational feature used other than its morse taper with non-indexed abutments Inherent *platform switching*

The rationale behind platform switching has varied in the literature. Many studies have theorized that an inflammatory infiltrate collects around the implant–abutment junction. By bringing this infiltrate medially, the inflammatory process is confined within the implant platform, thus lessening coronal bony resorption.

Maeda and colleagues (2008) theorized that the rationale behind platform switching was based on biomechanical advantages. They noted that platform switching not only decreased the stresses around the implant–abutment interface but also increased the forces around the abutment itself, which resulted in decreasing crestal bone loss.

Most studies, however, agree on one thing, the effectiveness of platform switching. Atieh's systematic review and meta-analysis in 2010 also validated this point. Atieh noted that the degree of crestal bone loss was affected by the difference between the diameter of the implant and the abutment. She noted a significant decrease in crestal bone resorption if the implant–abutment diameter difference was greater or equal to 0.4 mm.

Platform switching has been on the market since the introduction of the cone screw or morse taper designs with implants from companies such as Straumann, Ankylos, Bicon, or Astra. These conical designs have always inherently offered the benefits of platform switching.

COMPARISON OF DIFFERENT INTERNAL CONNECTION DESIGNS

As discussed earlier internal connection have several advantages over external connections, namely less screw loosening, improved esthetics, an advanced microbial seal, a strengthened implant–abutment joint connection, and a variety of options for platform switching. It is clear that practitioners and research, as well as manufacturers, are supporting the internal connection as the superior design. However, the internal connection market has splintered into several different competing designs. Little landmark research has been done to clarify which internal connection is likely to be the best design. The shear fact that the market has not rallied around one single internal connection type leads to the fact that solid research is still lacking.

There are advantages to having different internal implant connections on the market, but the decision between them is arguably more of a style or preference issue than anything else. This text certainly does not seek to endorse one connection design over another. Rather, this section characterizes the major friction-fit joints followed by the slip-fit joints currently available on the market (Table 4.1).

Friction-Fit Joints

Internal Hexagon and the Friction-Fit Joint

The internal hexagon connection has an internal hexagonal-shaped antirotational feature. Many implants utilizing the internal hex feature have moved away from the older slip-fit joint connections towards friction-fit joint connections. The friction between the abutment's tapered connection and the internal surface of the implant's connection creates the friction-fit joint. Since the abutment literally wedges into the implant's internal hex, the connection is called a "friction fit." This friction fit provides the microbial seal, minimizes the chance of screw loosening, and enhances joint stability with its internal connection.

Examples of internal hexagon friction-fit joint connections made by different manufacturers are discussed in this section.

Terminology

- *Friction-fit joint:* A connection feature where the mating components fit with friction rather than passivity
- *Butt joint:* The mating components of the abutment–implant interface consist of two right-angled surfaces
- *Beveled joint:* The mating components of the abutment–implant interface consist of beveled or angled joints
- *Internal hexagon or internal "hex":* An internal connection utilizing the hexagon as an antirotational feature internally within the implant

Zimmer Dental: Screw-Vent®   A prime example of an internal hexagon connection (Figure 4.3) with a friction-fit joint is the Screw-Vent joint connection used in Zimmer implants. This connection was initially conceived of by Dr Niznick in the 1980s and manufactured by Corevent Corporation. The design was later bought by Zimmer and is still used today.

In 1996, Binon and McHugh concluded that the rotational misfit for the Screw-Vent system used by Zimmer was 0 degrees when tightened to 30 N-cm. Under a scanning electron microscope, the abutment–implant interface reveals a virtual "cold weld" between the two surfaces. The 1.5 mm deep friction-fitting connection shields the screw from significant adverse tipping forces, preventing screw loosening.

BioHorizons   The internal connection made by BioHorizons can also be described as an internal hexagon friction-fit joint (Figure 4.4).

In a similar manner to the Screw-Vent joint, BioHorizonss also utilizes a 1.5 mm internal hex connection with a friction-fit joint. This abutment–implant interface creates a wedge effect, producing a seal.

Besides the friction-fit joint and internal connection, BioHorizons takes shielding the screw one step further with the use of the spiralock thread design. Spiralock technology is used in orthopedics and by aerospace industries to lessen screw loosening. With all the safeguards against screw loosening these designs nearly eliminate the problem of screw loosening.

Biomet 3i: Osseotite Certain™   The Biomet 3i connection (Figure 4.5) can also be classified as an internal hex

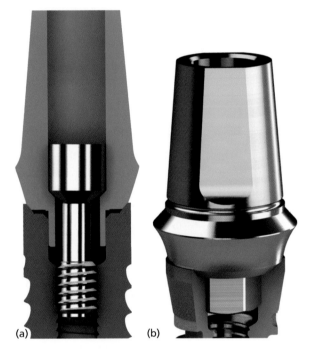

(a)   (b)

Figure 4.4   BioHorizons friction-fit internal hex connection. Courtesy of BioHorizons.

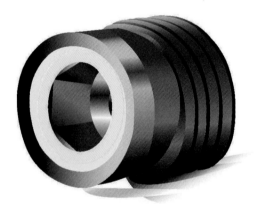

Figure 4.3   Screw-Vent friction-fit internal hex connection. Courtesy of Zimmer Dental. © 2012 Zimmer Dental, all rights reserved.

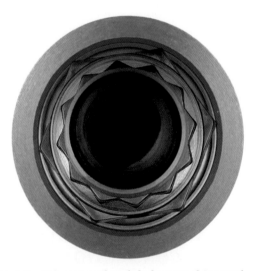

Figure 4.5   3i hexagonal and dodecagonal internal pattern. Courtesy of Biomet 3i. © 2009 Biomet 3i, all rights reserved.

connection consisting of a hexagonal and dodecagonal antirotational feature.

Biomet 3i's straight abutment utilizes the hexagon internal connection, while their 15-degree correctional abutments utilize the 12-point antirotational feature. This allows the positioning of the angled abutments to be placed at 30-degree intervals for an improved prosthetic position.

A unique feature with the 3i Osseotite Certain implant is that an audible "click" is heard when this abutment is fully seated. This enables a practitioner to be sure that a dental abutment is fully seated within its deep 4.0 mm internal engagement.

Unlike other internal hexagon connections, the 3i internal hexagon design also has the benefits of platform switching. In contrast to the cone screw and morse taper designs, where platform switching is an inherent property of the design, 3i's internal hexagon design (Figure 4.6) requires a narrower implant abutment on top of a widened implant platform.

Morse Taper and the Cone Screw

A morse taper is a cone within a cone. When two perfectly manufactured cones are tightly brought together, they provide a welded "friction-lock" stability. The degree of the morse taper is a percentage unit that reflects the shaft length relative to the radius of the shaft. For example, a 2% morse taper shaft length increase of 100 mm will have a radius increase of 2 mm. Whereas a 4% morse taper shaft length increase of 100 mm will have a radius increase of 4 mm. Most morse tapers vary from from 0% to 7%, but dentistry most commonly utilizes a 4–8% taper.

For clarity's sake this text will categorize a "true morse taper" connection as an implant system where an implant and abutment do not require an abutment screw between the two interfaces. The Bicon taper is a prime example of this. The term "cone screw" will be used for systems that utilize the benefits of the morse taper but connect the abutment to the implant with a retaining screw. There are multiple examples of the cone screw connection including those from Straumann, Astra, and Ankylos.

> **Terminology**
>
> - *True morse taper:* An abutment "cone within a cone" creating a seal between the implant and abutment without the need for a retaining screw
> - *Cone screw:* Internal, tapered, self-locking connection utilizing the self-locking principles of a morse taper but with a retaining screw connecting the abutment to the implant

Bicon: The True Morse Taper Bicon's implant–abutment connection is achieved with a 1.5-degree locking taper (Figure 4.7). The abutment is placed by tapping the abutment into the implant socket, which elastically deforms both the implant and abutment and is termed a "cold weld."

The advantage with using these implants is the fact that the abutment can fit anywhere in the 360 degrees of the implant. This allows the prosthesis to be positioned into an ideal orientation. Since there is no other

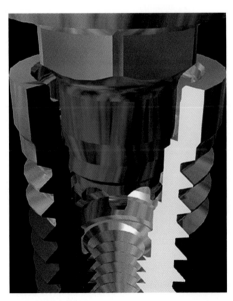

Figure 4.6 Biomet 3i internal hex connection. Courtesy of Biomet 3i. © 2009 Biomet 3i, all rights reserved.

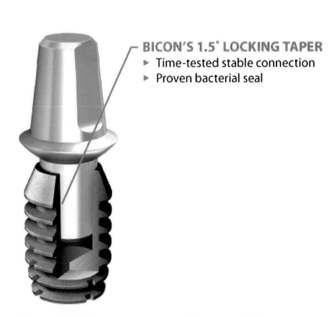

BICON'S 1.5° LOCKING TAPER
▸ Time-tested stable connection
▸ Proven bacterial seal

Figure 4.7 Bicon morse taper. Courtesy of Bicon.

implant system similar to that provided by Bicon, prosthetic options are limited to those offered by this company. The uniqueness of the system requires a learning curve for practitioners until they become comfortable with restoring this implant.

As outlined previously, Bicon has demonstrated the ability of their connection to provide an adequate microbial seal. The cold weld formed between the implant and abutment has been shown to create a hermetic seal keeping bacteria from colonizing the implant. In addition, the morse taper design naturally provides platform switching by medializing the implant–abutment connection.

Because there is no retaining screw with the Bicon system, there are no concerns about screw loosening. Generally in the posterior part of the mouth, occlusal forces decrease the preload of the retaining screw, but with the Bicon implant the occlusal forces strengthen the connection between the implant and abutment.

Removing a Bicon abutment from the implant requires the use of forceps to spin the abutment to overcome its cold weld with the implant.

Cone Screw

The cone screw utilizes similar principles to the morse taper. The cone within a cone connection provides a friction-lock connection, which is then retained with a screw. This morse taper friction lock not only provides a microbial seal but also antirotational features that ultimately reduce screw loosening. In addition, all cone screw connections inherently provide the benefits of platform switching.

Some cone screw connections utilize other antirotational features such as a hexagonal or dodecagonal feature, while others use the morse taper connection as the only antirotational feature. Leading cone screw implants on the market are provided by Straumann, Astra, and Ankylos.

Straumann Straumann's was the first cone screw attachment on the market with an 8-degree morse taper (Figure 4.8a). In addition, the synOcta™ attachment utilized by Straumann provides an internal octagon antirotational feature (Figure 4.8b) in combination with the morse taper connection.

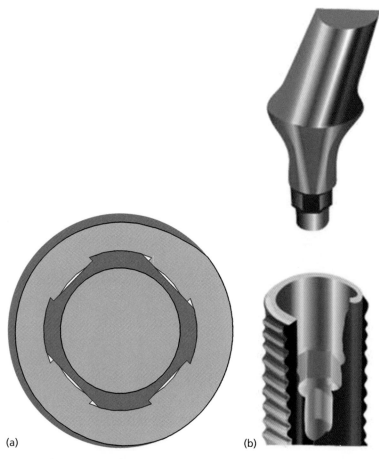

(a)   (b)

Figure 4.8 Straumann synOcta design. (a) 8-degree morse taper. (b) Internal antirotational feature. Courtesy of Straumann.

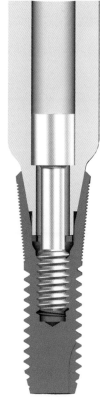

Figure 4.9 Astra cone screw connection. Courtesy of Astra Tech.

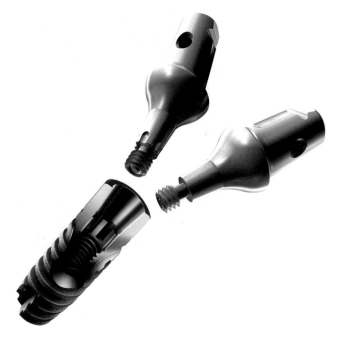

Figure 4.10 Ankylos cone screw connection. Courtesy of Dentsply (Ankylos).

Astra The Astra cone screw connection utilizes an 11-degree morse taper (Figure 4.9). In addition, the Astra implant also utilizes a dodecagonal antirotational feature in combination with the morse taper.

Ankylos Ankylos provides another common example of a cone screw connection with a 5.7-degree morse taper connection. This connection has indexed (Figure 4.10) and non-indexed abutment connections.

The non-indexed feature is truly a "cone within a cone," which uses the morse taper alone as an antirotational feature. This option has the additional benefit that the abutment can be connected in any position, which has an obvious prosthetic advantage.

Slip-fit Joints

Table 4.2 lists the different types of joints made by various manufacturers.

Internal Cylinder Hex

Another variant of the internal hexagon is the internal cylinder hexagon. Whereas standard internal hexagon joints have their hex joint nearly 1.5 mm deep, this connection has the hex joint up to 5 mm deep within the implant. The most popular internal

Table 4.2 Slip-fit joint connections

Company	Connection	Unique features
Frialit-2	Internal cylinder hex	Deep internal connection
Neoss	Spline connection	Potential for platform switching
Camlog	Cam-tube connection	Deepest, most stable internal connection
Nobel	Tri-channel or tri-lobed connection	1.2 mm deep internal connection
Keystone	Six-lobed connection	Variant of the tri-lobe

cylinder hexagon joint is not a friction-fit joint but rather a slip-fit joint. The major advantage of this connection is that the deep 5 mm connection provides a significantly superior joint strength in comparison with the external connection.

Mollersten et al. (1997) plainly showed that deep joints are more likely to resist bending forces than shallow joints. This connection capitalizes on this concept.

Terminology

- *Internal cylinder hex:* A cylindrical abutment with a deep 5 mm internal implant–abutment hex connection, which is connected to the implant via a retaining screw
- *Slip-fit joint:* The implant–abutment connection has a passive fit between the two mating connections

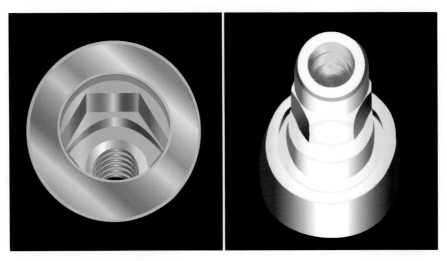

Figure 4.11 Frialit-2 internal cylinder connection.

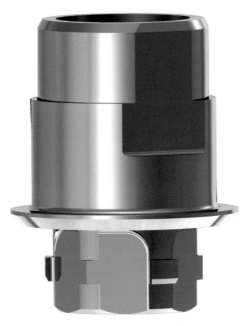

Figure 4.12 Neoss abutment with a spline connection. Courtesy of Neoss. © 2010 Neoss, all rights reserved.

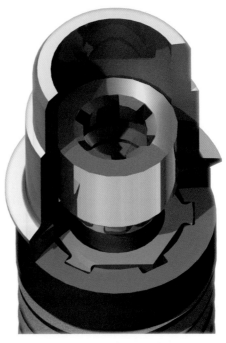

Figure 4.13 Neoss spline connection. Courtesy of Neoss. © 2010 Neoss, all rights reserved.

The Frialit-2 is an example of an internal cylinder hex with a 5 mm deep internal hex connection and a slip-fit joint (Figure 4.11).

Spline Connections

The spline connection utilizes keys or "splines" (Figure 4.12) to connect the implant and abutment through grooves in a slip-fit joint. There are few data on this connection type since only a few implant companies use this technique. Neoss is one of the companies with spline connection.

Terminology

- *Spline:* Six parallel keys or "splines" alternate with six grooves connecting the implant and the abutment together (both external and internal connections have utilized splines)

Neoss The internal spline connection of the Neoss implant is called Neolinks (Figure 4.13). This connection ensures precision of fit, limits micro-motion, and provides load relief to the screw. It has a narrower

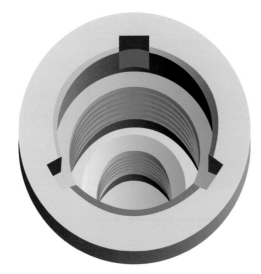

Figure 4.14 Camlog's cam tube connection. Courtesy of Camlog.

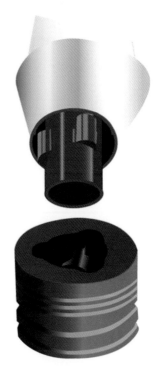

Figure 4.15 Nobel Biocare tri-channel design.

abutment than its implant platform, providing benefits of platform switching.

Cam Tube and Tri-Channel Connections

The deep cam tube and tri-channel connections utilize three deep internal connecting engagements in a slip-fit joint (Figure 4.14).

The deep cam tube has been defined as a "tube-in-tube" slip-fit joint. The cam tube connection has the deepest and strongest internal connection on the market, with a 5.4 mm deep internal connection. Due to the stability of the joint there is minimal screw loosening. In addition, the deep connection provides a superb microbial seal. The cam tube connection is utilized by the Camlog implant company.

The tri-channel or "tri-lobe" connection from Nobel Biocare (Figure 4.15) has a close similiarity to the cam tube connection (Figure 4.16). This connection utilizes a tri-channel with a 1.2 mm depth slip-fit joint.

The keystone connection (Figure 4.17) is a modified version of the tri-channel connection. It offers a six-lobed rather than a three-lobed approach to the internal connection.

Terminology

- *Cam tube:* Tube-in-tube abutment connection where three cam tubes are seated within the body of the implant
- *Tri-channel or tri-lobed design:* Three lateral channels project from the abutment into the implant body

Connection Diversification among Implant Companies

It is important to note that although implant companies originally were known for a single connection design, this is certainly not the case today. For instance, 3i not only has an internal hex and external hex but has also introduced the Osseotite TG, which utilizes a cone screw connection comparable to that from Straumann.

Implant Direct offers an internal hex (similar to BioHorizonss or Zimmer), an internal octagon (similar to Straumann), as well as an internal tri-lobe (comparable to Nobel Biocare). Southern implants utilize an internal octagon (similar to Straumann) as well as a tri-lobe connection (similar to Nobel Biocare). Even Nobel Biocare has diversified from their tri-lobe connection into offering a conical connection.

Since most of the connection patents have ended implant companies are diversifying their abutment connections by copying each other.

CONCLUSIONS

In conclusion, implant–abutment connections have progressed from the early external hex connection to more advanced internal connections. The internal connection is clearly a superior design to the external one and the market is shifting more towards the use

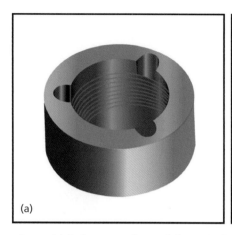
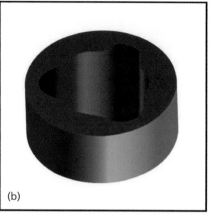

(a)   (b)

Figure 4.16   Comparison of (a) the cam tube and (b) a tri-channel connection.

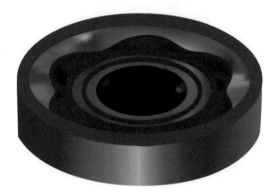

Figure 4.17   Keystone connection.

of internal connections with deep internal joints. Among the several designs available, the market has not rallied around one but rather has branched out into several varying options. Each system has the inherent advantages found with internal connections, although there is no solidifying evidence pointing to a single best internal connection type.

Initially, each dental implant company was isolated with differing patented abutment connection designs. More recently, several companies have diversified the abutment connections they offer. With this diversification within each company further unbiased research will undoubtedly develop. The future appears bright with upcoming research directing the market towards a clinically proven favorable internal connection design.

REFERENCES AND ADDITIONAL READING

Atieh, M.A. (2010). Platform switching for marginal bone preservation around dental implants: a systematic review and meta-analysis. *Journal of Periodontology*, 81(10), 1350–1366.

Babbush, C. (2005). Evolution of a dental implant practice: the camlog implant system. *New York State Dental Journal*, 71(6), 24–31.

Barbosa, G.S., Bernardes, S.R., Neves, F.D., Fernandes Neto, A.J., Mattos, M.D., & Ribeiro, R.F. (2008). Relation between implant/abutment vertical misfit and torque loss of abutment screws. *Brazilian Dental Journal*, 19(4), 458–463.

Baumgarten, H., Cocchetto, R., Testori, T., Meltzer, A., & Porter, S. (2005). A new implant design for crestal bone preservation: initial observations and case report. *Practical Procedures and Aesthetic Dentistry*, 17, 735–740.

Becker, W. & Becker, B. (1995). Replacement of maxillary and mandibular molars with single endosseous implant restorations: a retrospective study. *Journal of Prosthetic Dentistry*, 74(1), 51–55.

Binon, P. (1995). Evaluation of machining accuracy and consistency of selected implants,standard abutments, and laboratory analogs. *International Journal of Prosthodontics*, 8, 162–178.

Binon, P. (2000). Implants and components: entering the new millennium. *International Journal of Oral and Maxillofacial Implants*, 15(1), 76–94.

Binon, P. & McHugh, M. (1996). The effect of eliminating implant/abutment rotational misfit on screw joint stability. *International Journal of Prosthodontics*, 9(6), 511–519.

Bozkaya, D. & Müftü, S. (2003). Mechanics of the taper integrated screwed-in (tis) abutments used dental implants. *Journal of Biometrics*, 38(1), 87–97.

Broggini, N., McManus, L., Hermann, J., et al. (2006). Peri-implant inflammation defined by the implant-abutment interface. *Journal of Dental Research*, 85(5), 473–478.

Cappiello, M., Luongo, R., Di Iorio, D., Bugea, C., Cocchetto, R., & Celletti, R. (2008). Evaluation of peri-implant bone loss around platform-switched implants. *International Journal of Periodontics and Restorative Dentistry*, 28, 347–355.

Carrilho, G., Dias, R., & Elias, C. (2005). Comparison of external and internal hex implants' rotational freedom: a pilot study. *International Journal of Prosthodontics*, 18(2), 165–166.

Coelho, P.G., Sudack, P., Suzuk, M., Kurtz, K.S., Romanos, G.E., & Silva, N. (2008). In vitro evaluation of the implant abutment connection sealing capability of different implant systems. *Journal of Oral Rehabilitation*, 35, 917–924.

Dibart, S., Warbington, M., Fan Su, M., & Skobe, Z. (2004). Elongation and preload stress in dental implant abutment screws. Poster presented at the American Academy of Periodontology.

Dibart, S., Warbington, M., Fan Su, M., & Skobe, Z. (2005). In vitro evaluation of the implant-abutment bacterial seal: the locking taper system. *International Journal of Oral and Maxillofacial Implants*, 20(5), 732–737.

Finger, I.M., Castellon, P., Block, M., & Elian, N. (2003). The evolution of external and internal implant/abutment connections. *Practical Procedures and Aesthetic Dentistry*, 15(8th series), 625–632.

Gardner, D.M. (2005). Platform switching as a means to achieving implant esthetics. *New York State Dental Journal*, 71(3), 34–37.

Ha, C., Kim, C., Lim, Y., & Jang, K. (2005). The effect of internal implant–abutment connection and diameter on screw loosening. *Journal of the Korean Academy of Prosthodontics*, 43(3), 379–392.

Haack, J., Sakaquchi, R., Sun, T., & Coffey, J. (1995). Elongation and preload stress in dental implant abutment screws. *International Journal of Oral and Maxillofacial Implants*, 10(5), 529–536.

Harder, S., Dimaczek, B., Acil, Y., Terheyden, H., Freitag-Wolf, S., & Kern, M. (2009). Molecular leakage at implant-abutment connection – in vitro investigation of tightness of internal conical implant–abutment connections against endotoxin penetration. *Clinical Oral Investigations*, 14(4), 427–432.

Hurzeler, M., Fickl, S., Zuhr, O., & Wachtel, H. (2007). Peri-implant bone level around implants with platform-switched abutments: preliminary data from a prospective study. *Journal of Oral and Maxillofacial Surgery*, 65(7), 33–39.

Jemt, T., Laney, W., Harris, D., et al. (1991). Osseointegrated implants for single tooth replacement: a 1-year report from a multicenter prospective study. *International Journal of Oral and Maxillofacial Implants*, 6(1), 29–36.

Jemt, T., Linden, B., & Lekholm, U. (1992). Failures and complications in 127 consecutively inserted fixed prosthesis supported by Branemark implants: from prostheses treatment to first annual check up. *Journal of Oral and Maxillofacial Implants*, 7(1), 40–44.

Jemt, T., & Pettersson, P. (1993). A 3-year follow-up study on single implant treatment. *Journal of Dentistry*, 21(4), 203–208.

Khraisat, A., Baqain, Z.H., Smadi, L., Nomura, S., Miyakawa, O., & Elnasser, Z. (2006). Abutment rotational displacement of external hexagon implant system under lateral cyclic loading. *Clinical Implant Dentistry and Related Research*, 8(2), 95–99.

Laney, W., Jemt, T., Harris, D., & Krogh, P. (1994). Osseointegrated implants for single-tooth replacement: progress report from a multicenter prospective study after 3 years. *International Journal of Oral and Maxillofacial Implants*, 9(1), 49–54.

Lazzara, R. & Porter, S. S. (2006). Platform switching: a new concept in implant dentistry for controlling postrestora-tive crestal bone levels. *International Journal of Periodontics and Restorative Dentistry*, 26, 9–17.

Lee, T., Han, J., Yang, J., Lee, J., & Kim, S. (2008). The assessment of abutment screw stability between the external and internal hexagonal joint under cyclic loading. *Journal of the Korean Academy of Prosthodontics*, 46(6), 561.

Levine, R., Clem, D., Wilson, T., Higginbottom, F., & Solnit, G. (1999). Multicenter retrospective analysis of the ITI implant system used for single-tooth replacements: results of loading for 2 or more years. *International Journal of Oral and Maxillofacial Implants*, 14(4), 516–520.

Luongo, R., Traini, T., Guidone, P.C., Bianco, G., Cocchetto, R., & Celletti, R. (2008). Hard and soft tissue responses to the platform-switching technique. *International Journal of Periodontics and Restorative Dentistry*, 28, 551.

Maeda, Y., Horisaka, M., & Yagi, K. (2008). Biomechanical rationale for a single implant-retained mandibular over-denture: an in vivo study. *Clinical Oral Implants Research*, 19, 271–275.

Mairgünther, R. & Netwig, G. (1992). Das Dichtigkeits-verhalten des Verbindungssystems beim zweiphasigen Ankylos-Implantat [The tightness behavior of the connection system of the 2-phase Ankylos implant]. *Zeitschrift für Zahnärztliche Implantologie*, V, 50–53.

Meng, J., Everts, J., Qian, F., & Gratton, D. (2007). Influence of connection geometry on dynamic micromotion at the implant–abutment interface. *International Journal of Prosthodontics*, 20(6), 623–625.

Miloro, M., Ghali, G.E., Larsen, P.E., & Waite, P. (2004). *Peterson's Principles of Oral and Maxillofacial Surgery*. Hamilton, Ontario: BC Decker.

Mollersten, L., Lockowandt, P., & Linden, L. (1997). Comparison of strength and failure mode of seven implant systems: an in vitro test. *Journal of Prosthetic Dentistry*, 78(6), 582–591.

Narang, P., Gupta, H., Arora, A., & Bhandari, A. (2011). Biomechanics of implant abutment connection: a review. *Indian Journal of Stomatology*, 2(2), 108–112.

Norton, M.R. (1997). An in vitro evaluation of the strength of an internal conical interface compared to a butt joint interface in implant design. *Clinical Oral Implants Research*, 8(4), 290–298.

Norton, M.R. (2000). In vitro evaluation of the strength of the conical implant-to-abutment joint in two commercially available implant systems. *Journal of Prosthetic Dentistry*, 83(5), 567–571.

Prasad, K.D., Shetty, M., Bansal, N., & Hegde, C. (2011). Platform switching: an answer to crestal bone loss. *Journal of Dental Implants*, 1(1), 13–17.

Quek, H.C., Tan, K.B., & Nicholls, J. (2008). Load fatigue performance of four implant–abutment interface designs: effect of torque level and implant system. *Journal of Prosthetic Dentistry*, 100(1), 73–73.

Ricomini Filho, A.P., Fernandes, F.F., Straioto, F.G., Silva, W.D., & Del Bel Cury, A.A. (2010). Preload loss and bacterial penetration on different implant–abutment connection systems. *Brazilian Dental Journal*, 21(2), 123–129.

Schrotenboer, J., Tsao, Y., Kinariwala, V., & Wang, H. (2009). Effect of platform switching on implant crest bone stress: a finite element analysis. *Implant Dentistry*, 18(3), 260–269.

Segundo, R., Oshima, H., Silva, I., Júnior, L., Mota, E., & Coelho, L. (2007). Stress distribution on external hexagon implant system using 3D finite element analysis. *Acta Odontológica Latinoamicana*, 20, 2nd series, 79–81.

Semper, W., Kraft, S., Krüger, T., & Nelson, K. (2009). Theoretical considerations: implant positional index design. *Journal of Dental Research*, 88(8), 725–730.

Sethi, A. & Kaus, T. (2002). *An implant that does not smell: the Ankylos implant*. http://www.implantynacalezycie.pl/artykuly/An%20implant%20that%20doesn't%20smell.pdf (last accessed April 2014).

Steinebrunner, L., Wolfart, S., Bobmann, K., & Kern, M. (2005). In vitro evaluation of bacterial leakage along the implant abutment–interface of different implant systems. *International Journal of Oral and Maxillofacial Implants*, 20, 875–881.

Theoharidou, A., Petridis, H., Tzannas, K., & Garefis, P. (2008). Abutment screw loosening in single-implant restorations: a systematic review. *International Journal of Oral and Maxillofacial Implants*, 23(4), 681–690.

Urdaneta, R.A. & Marincola, M. (2007). The integrated abutment crown, a screwless and cementless restoration for single-tooth implants: a report on a new technique. *Journal of Prosthodontics*, 16(4), 311–318.

Vigolo, P., Odont, Fonzi, F., Majzoub, Z., & Cordioli, G. (2005). An in vitro evaluation of ZiReal abutments with hexagonal connection: in original state and following abutment preparation. *International Journal of Oral and Maxillofacial Implants*, 20(1), 108–114.

Weinberg, L. (1993). The biomechanics of force distribution in implant-supported prostheses. *International Journal of Oral and Maxillofacial Implants*, 8(1), 19–31.

Zarb, G., & Schmitt, A. (1990). The longitudinal clinical effectiveness of osseointegrated dental implants: the Toronto study. Part I: Surgical results. *Journal of Prosthetic Dentistry*, 63(4), 451–457.

5

Prefabricated Implant Abutments

Paul P. Binon

Department of Restorative Dentistry, University of California at San Francisco, CA; Graduate Prosthodontics, Indiana University, Indianapolis, IN; and Private Practice, Roseville, CA

INTRODUCTION

Over the past 35 years the number and variety of prefabricated implant abutments has increased significantly. Short span and single teeth replacements with Branemark implants were first reported by Jemt in 1986 using modified abutments. In the same year Sullivan (1986) and Krogh (1986) each published independent papers on treating partially edentulous areas with fixed implants supported prosthesis. This chapter starts with a historical account of the development of prefabricated implant abutments.

CHRONOLOGICAL DEVELOPMENT OF PREFABRICATED ABUTMENTS

The original Branemark abutment was a hollow cylinder with a mated internal hexagonal that fixed over the top of the implant and projected through the soft tissue and was secured with an abutment screw that was tightened into place. This "standard" abutment, also know as a "flat top," came in a variety of heights and was primarily intended to support a hybrid fixed denture. The prosthesis design incorporated machined gold cylinders that were cast as part of a metal framework intended to receive porcelain that fitted intimately against the standard abutment and was held in place with gold prosthetic screws.

Historically, the first fixed, partial denture, cementable abutment designs were threaded tapered posts that screwed into the body of the dental implant. Manu-

facturers such as Core-Vent, Calcitek, and Implant Innovations introduced one-piece screw-in abutments to secure cemented crowns and bridges (Niznick and Misch 1988). These components were hand tightened or ratcheted into the threaded recessed area within the implant. Initial designs had no antirotational element incorporated. Some manufacturers did incorporate thread timing so that, if an indexing flat was incorporated on the post, the same orientation could be achieved repeatedly. The post could be modified inside or outside of the mouth to correct minor angulation changes and vertical height modifications. Perfect realignment and orientation was often difficult with these designs and abutment loosening did occur.

Another early approach was to cement the abutment post into a recess within the implant body (Niznick and Misch 1988). Additional modification led to a combination threaded/cementable recess within the implant body. The neck of some of the abutment posts had a smaller diameter waist that would allow bending to alter head angulation. This offered some challenges if the abutment came loose and had to be re-cemented or had to be removed if the neck of the abutment fractured.

Some implant companies created additional "standard" abutments with shorter length sleeves that could be used for crown and bridge applications. Even with these additional components, crown and bridge applications were severely limited from an esthetic standpoint. Since the platform size of the screw in abutment typically matched that of the implant, the resulting emergence profile of the metal-ceramic restoration did not replicate that of a natural tooth. Considerable efforts, however, were made by many clinicians and technicians to overcome this liability with custom milled bars, substructures, and metal-ceramic superstructures.

A significant breakthrough occurred with the development of the plastic UCLA abutment (Lewis et al. 1988, 1992). This design eliminated the need for an intervening component since it engaged the implant hexagonal interface directly. Initially it consisted of a plastic sleeve that could be modified with wax and cast in metal-ceramic to support the porcelain. The component also had a larger securing screw that resisted much higher bending loads. Multiple implant supporting units could be incorporated into a metal-ceramic fixed partial denture (FPD) with a more pleasing natural emergence profile and greater resistance to loosening. The biggest disadvantage of the abutment was the inherent casting error at the implant–abutment interface (Kan et al. 1999; Silveira et al. 2002).

The next logical step occurred when a UCLA-type sleeve was prefabricated into a metal chimney abutment with multiple flats. It served as a stand-alone abutment that would accommodate a PFM-cemented restoration. The resulting restoration has a more acceptable emergence profile and no screw access hole to compromise the occlusal surface. Another significant advantage of the stock preformed metal abutments over the castable plastic abutments is the improved implant–abutment interface fit. This design led others to follow suit with more prosthetic-friendly designs that incorporated slight tapers (2 to 5 degrees) (Byrne et al. 1998).

Clinicians and manufacturers soon recognized that abutments that allowed angulation changes were a necessity (Drago 1991). Implant systems with antirotational implant–abutment interfaces introduced two-piece abutments consisting of an abutment fastening screw and an angled clinical abutment component that changed direction from the long axis of the implant to a specified angle offset. This is most helpful in the maxillary arch where the incisor root axis is at about 60 degrees with the horizontal plane and progresses with a less acute angle posteriorly to the second molar (Chandra et al. 2008).

Since the placement of an implant typically follows the central axis of the alveolar process, the projected implant axis would penetrate the facial or buccal aspect of the clinical crowns. To avoid this, abutments with angulation offsets are available ranging from 12 to 30 degrees. In most instances the prefabricated abutments would still require some modification. Typically it involves a reduction in height and modification of the wall alignment with adjacent abutments to facilitate draw. Initially, the angled abutment could be rotated to six different rotational locations on the hexagonal. Additional rotational capability was made available in some systems by doubling the hexagonal indexing points within the recess, allowing 12 different rotational locations on the implant hex.

With the advent of internal connections, the specific engagement design, be it an internal hexagonal or tri-lobed design, dictates the specific rotational offset.

In addition to incorporating angulation changes, a cervical collar was added to virtually all the prefabricated abutments that allowed for a change in emergence profile. The angulated abutment typically requires an abutment cervical collar that is narrow on the facial and taller on the lingual to accommodate the change in the clinical crowns engagement angle. A variety of collar heights are typically available permitting selection based on mucosal thickness. Also incorporated into the vertical part of most of the abutments is an indexing flat that makes orientation of the crown much easier.

Recent Developments

Today, virtually all of the implant manufactures provide angulation correction abutments in their product line. Depending on the manufacturer, both straight and angled abutments may have straight or flared walls to offset the round implant loading platform and to provide a better emergence profile for the crown restoration. The shoulder of the abutment may also be contoured, changing from a minimal height on the facial to a higher lingual height. A few manufacturers have also increased the facial/lingual width to more closely emulate the ovoid/triangular shape of most teeth in the cervical area. In an effort to have less graying discoloration through thin facial tissues, some manufacturers have gold-colored or light pink-colored abutment surfaces.

One manufacturer has incorporated the implant mount and a temporary cylinder into one integrated unit. The clinician upon placement of the implant into the osteotomy can remove the upper segment and cut off the implant mount and use the lower half of the mount as a temporary cylinder to fabricate a temporary restoration.

More recent advances have been made with the design of posterior abutments. Several manufactures have prefabricated abutments that emulate natural tooth preparations. They typically come available in two heights and three or more collar heights ranging from 0.5 to 3 mm. Examples of these innovative products are the Easy Abutments™ by Nobel Biocare and the Express Abutments™ by Neoss. Corresponding impression components and plastic burn-out casting sleeves, along with healing cap are available and are usually packaged and sold as a unit. Once the abutment has been placed on the implant, the remaining treatment sequence corresponds to that of a conventional crown and bridge. In select posterior cases where this applies, it is cost effective and saves the clinician time with respect to selecting and ordering components.

In comparing costs, prefabricated abutments range from US$85 to $250 depending on the implant system. Laboratory charges for custom zirconium abutments (Atlantis™) currently run at $350 per unit. Custom gold abutments approximate the same cost, depending on the current price of the gold alloy. Laboratory charges for modifications to prefabricated abutments run from no charge to $50 per unit depending on the degree of modification.

Recent histologic evaluation of micro-grooved roughened surfaces (Laser-Lok™ by BioHorizons) on the coronal portion of dental implants have demonstrated connective tissue attachment that emulates sharpey fibers (Nevins et al. 2008). Such a connection inhibits epithelial downgrowth and potentially preserves the coronal bone level and establishes a zone of "biologic width." Subsequent investigations demonstrated a connective tissue attachment to Laser-Microgrooved Abutments as part of a human histologic study. The clinical question as to what to expect when the healing abutment was to be replaced with a permanent abutment was unanswered. At that time, a continuation of the study replaced the healing abutment with a two-piece permanent abutment. That abutment was later biopsied with the surrounding soft tissue to demonstrate that the apical migration of the epithelium was inhibited after the abutment transfer. The same laser surface has been added to prefabricated abutments (Nevins et al. 2010). The protocol calls for seating the abutment at the time of implant insertion and without disruption during the life of the restoration. Having a soft tissue attachment on the abutment and implant may provide even greater protection for the osseous structures and greater resistance to mechanical and inflammatory insults (Geurs et al. 2011; Nevins et al. 2012).

The increased popularity of implant-supported dentistry in the esthetic area raised concerns of visible discoloration resulting from the titanium metallic color showing through thin gingival tissues (Glauser et al. 2004). Furthermore, greater use of all-ceramic restorations resulted in a need for an abutment that did not diminish their natural translucency and vitality (Heydecke et al. 2002). As an alternative to titanium abutments, all-ceramic abutments were introduced in 1993 (Andersson et al. 2001). These initial non-metallic abutments were made of sintered aluminum oxide (Al_2O_3).

Soon after, zirconium oxide abutments were introduced (Piconi and Maccauro 1999). Alumina abutments were prone to micro-crack propagation during preparation, resulting in fractures (Kucey and Fraser 2000; Watkin and Kerstein 2008). This inherent weakness was overcome by the tougher mechanical proper-

ties of zirconium (Presipino and Ingber 1993). Zirconia also has greater radio-opacity than its aluminum oxide counterpart. The latter, however, is still preferred when thin facial tissue presents in high lip line patients. The cumulative success rate of both materials at 5 to 10 years is reported at 97% (Andersson et al. 2003).

There is no question that prefabricated abutments offer several advantages, including cost. Prefabricated components are easy to use and reduce the laboratory expenses involved in crown and bridge applications. The main difficulty, however, lies with the diameter of the loading platform and the resulting emergence profile. With custom abutments, the transition from the implant to the cervical area of the crown is better controlled. The custom abutment reduces the abruptness of the angulation transition and can be modified to emulate the cross-sectional anatomy of the root at the cervical area. Efforts to overcome this limitation by using an expanding collar flare have improved the emergence profile but it does not always eliminate the entire problem, especially in the anterior esthetic zone. Less critical is the posterior area. Hence prefab abutments have the best application in that area of the mouth. For optimal esthetics, custom abutments should be used in the esthetic zone.

EXAMPLES OF PREFABRICATED ABUTMENTS

Biomet 3i straight and pre-angled abutments (Figure 5.1) can be altered with rotary instruments in the

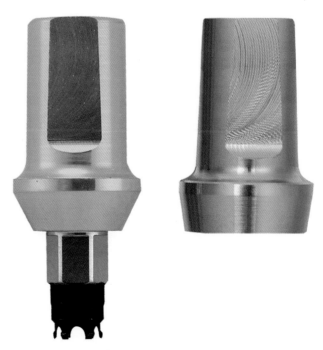

Figure 5.1 Straight and pre-angled GingiHue® Abutments. Courtesy of Biomet 3i.

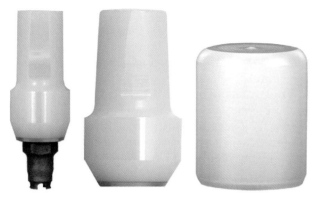

Figure 5.2 Straight and pre-angled ZiReal Abutments. Courtesy of Biomet 3i.

mouth or mounted on an abutment holder. The gold-colored GingiHue® Abutment is intended to mask gray penetration through the gingival tissues.

The ZiReal® Abutment (Figure 5.2) is a non-metalic abutment designed for use with all-ceramic restorations. Once seated in the mouth, the abutments can be treated as conventional crown and bridge preparations.

Astra abutments (Figures 5.3 and 5.4) are unique in having indexed, tapered, conical connections. They offer straight, angled, and contoured abutments in zirconia and titanium. The shoulders can be modified to a limited extent.

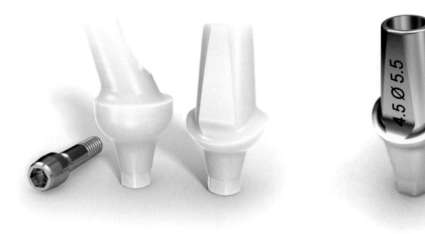

Figure 5.3 Astra zirconia and titanium abutments. Courtesy of Dentsply (Astra).

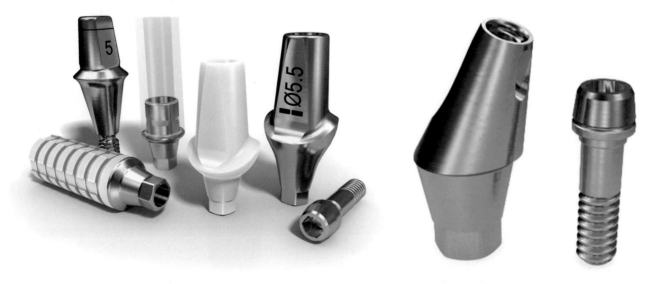

Figure 5.4 Astra angled and straight cervical contoured abutments. Courtesy of Dentsply (Astra).

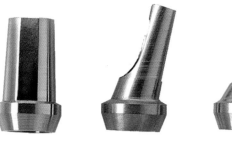

Figure 5.5 Keystone straight and angled cuff titanium abutments. Courtesy of Keystone Dental.

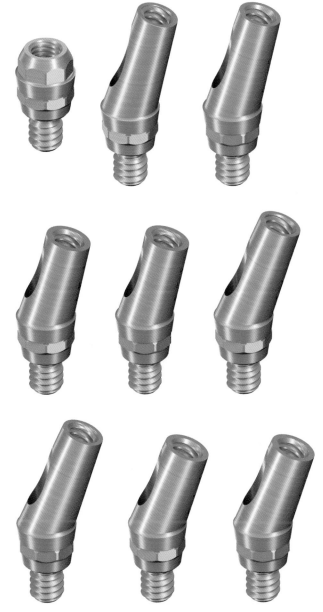

Figure 5.6 Straumann angled titanium abutments intended for cemented crown and bridge applications. Courtesy of Straumann.

Virtually all the implant companies fabricate titanium abutments with slight variations in the cervical design. The Keystone (formerly Lifecore) abutment has a narrower shoulder with a straight wall (Figure 5.5). This applies to both the straight and angled titanium abutments.

Conversely, the Straumann abutments illustrated in Figure 5.6 have essentially no machined shoulder. The implant crown is often seated to the flared shoulder of the implant.

Straumann also has all-inclusive kits (Figure 5.7) available that include an abutment, impression transfer coping, analog, and protective cap for implant-supported fixed crown and bridge applications.

Most of the implant manufacturers offer more scalloped shoulder designs as illustrated by the Neoss titanium abutments (Figure 5.8).

Hex-Lock™ abutments by Zimmer (Figure 5.9) are available in a variety of implant platforms (3.4, 4.5, and 5.7 mm), which is typical of most manufacturers. It also has an emergence profile with a wider cervical crown diameter for a more natural crown width.

The Genesis implant system (Figure 5.10) by Keystone offers consistent contours for all of its components, a six-lobed implant–abutment connection and a light pink color to mask metallic blush through thin gingival tissues.

Implant Direct Sybron Int. (Figure 5.11) implant systems (Legacy™, Tri-Lobe, Spectra-System®, RePlant®, Swish Plus™) incorporate a carrier and a temporary or prep-able abutment attached to the implant.

Once the implant has been fully seated in the osteotomy, the transfer/carrier can be used as a closed tray impression coping. Another option is to remove the carrier screw and cut the colored prescored section of the carrier/transfer and use it as a temporary abutment. The system is well designed for optimal utilization and minimal additional expense.

BioHorizons (Figure 5.12) has introduced prefabricated abutments with Laser-Lok micro-channels that encourage bone and connective tissue attachment. The abutment is intended to be seated at the time of implant placement and to remain undisturbed through the final restoration.

A comparison between conventional implant/abutments and Laser-Lok implant/abutments at a microscopic level documents the preserved bone height and connective tissue attachment (Figure 5.13).

Progressively higher magnification images of the Laser-Lok micro-channels confirm the attachment of collagen fibers, creating a mucosal barrier or biologic width preventing the downgrowth of epithelium (Figure 5.14).

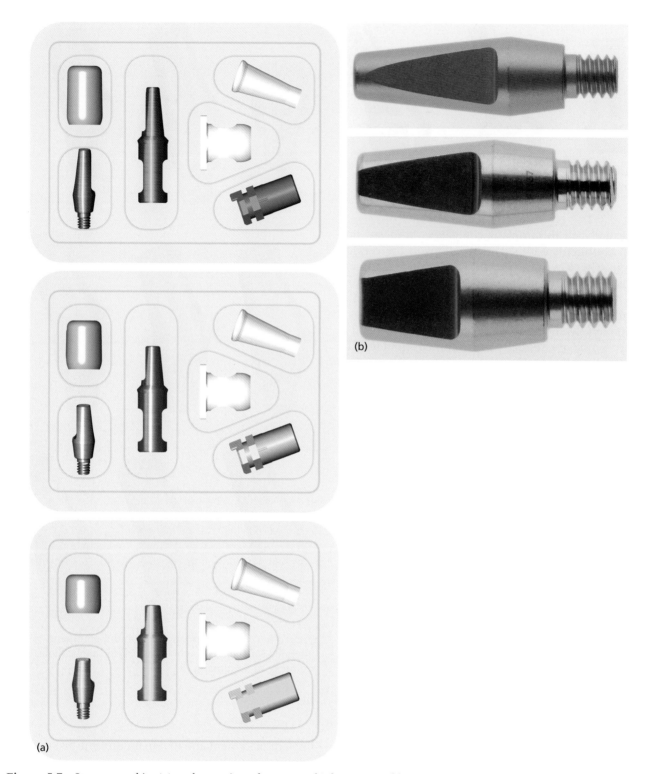

Figure 5.7 Straumann kits (a) and one-piece abutments (b) for cementable restorations. Courtesy of Straumann.

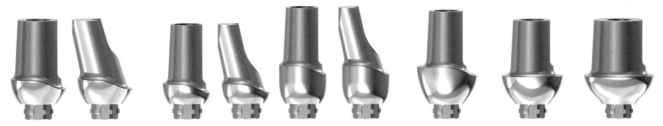

Figure 5.8 Neoss straight and angled titanium abutments. Courtesy of Neoss.

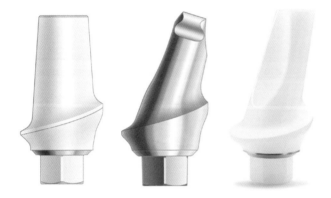

Figure 5.9 Examples of Zimmer prefabricated straight and angled abutments. Courtesy of Zimmer Dental.

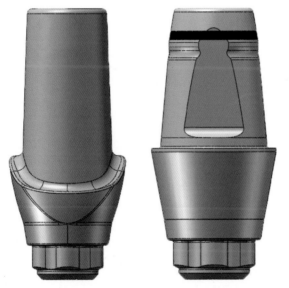

Figure 5.10 Genesis abutments from Keystone offer an elongated buccolingual oval circumference with a scalloped shoulder design as well as the classic round design. Courtesy of Keystone Dental.

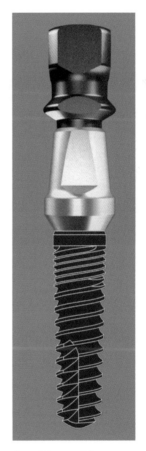

Figure 5.11 Implant Direct with a premounted carrier, transfer, and final abutment mounted to the implant. Courtesy of Implant Direct.

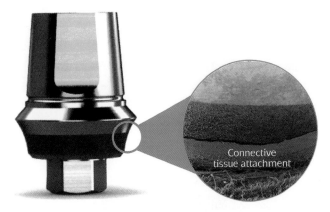

Figure 5.12 Laser-Lok abutment with micro-channels. Courtesy of Biohorizons.

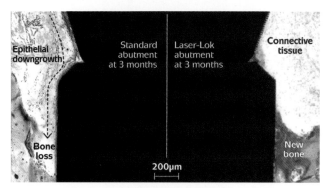

Figure 5.13 Cross-sectional magnification showing the soft tissue adaptation providing a mucosal barrier. Source: Nevins, M., Kim, D.M., Jun, S.H., Guze, K., Schupbach, P., & Nevins, M.L. (2010). Histologic evidence of a connective tissue attachment to laser microgrooved abutments: a canine study. *International Journal of Periodontics and Restorative Dentistry*, 30, 245–255.

CLINICAL EXAMPLES

Some clinical examples of prefabricated cases are presented in the figures that accompany this text. They offer progressive steps in the use of selected abutments that are generally representative of what is currently available. A wide variety of abutment designs and features are available today. Some typical variations offered by a number of manufacturers are illustrated at the end of this chapter. It is hoped that the information presented in this chapter, the clinical cases documented, and illustrations presented, will aid the clinician in making prudent choices related to available systems and their components.

Nobel Biocare Prefabricated Abutment: Single Tooth Replacement

The procedure for the placement of a single implant with a prefabricated Nobel Biocare 4.3 mm diameter Easy Abutment is shown in Figure 5.15.

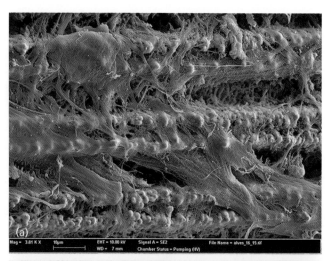

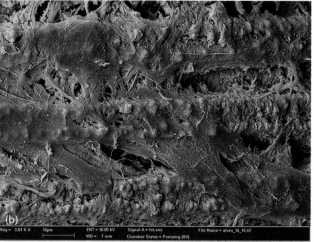

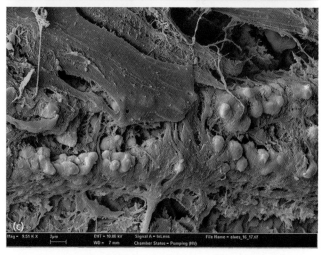

Figure 5.14 Scanning electron microscope images documenting collagen fiber attachment into the microgrooves, with (a) and (b) at a lower magnification than (c). Courtesy of BioHorizons. Nevins, M., Nevins, M.L., Camelo, M., Boyesen, J.L., & Kim, D.M. (2008). Human histologic evidence of a connective tissue attachment to a dental implant. *International Journal of Periodontics and Restorative Dentistry*, 28, 111–121.

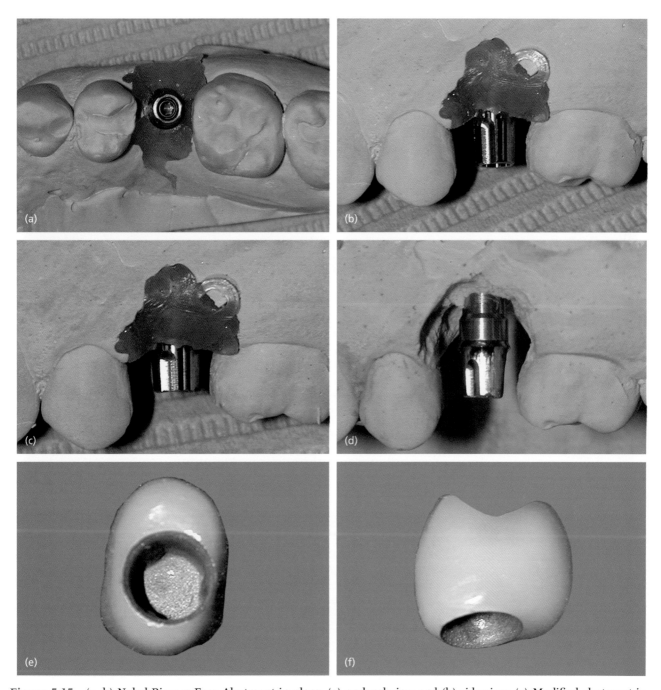

Figure 5.15 (a, b) Nobel Biocare Easy Abutment in place: (a) occlusal view and (b) side view. (c) Modified abutment in place with adequate occlusal clearance. (d) Clearer view of the entire abutment showing that sufficient vertical height remains to retain a cemented crown restoration. (e, f) Completed restoration showing the orientation groove and near parallel walls for optimal retention: (e) internal view and (f) proximal view.

The abutment may need to be altered to allow for additional occlusal clearance. The abutment is marked with a fine-tip indelible marker and removed from the model and attached to an analog. A high speed diamond cutter can easily remove the necessary material for appropriate clearance. It is quite typical for prefabricated abutments to require some modification. Slight alterations in height and angulation are still more cost effective than custom cast or milled abutments. The abutment needs to have sufficient vertical height to retain a cemented crown restoration.

The completed restoration has an orientation groove and near parallel walls for optimal retention. There may be limitations when using a prefabricated abutment in altering the crown to abutment contours, while a custom abutment allows the correction of both the buccolingual and proximal crown contours. The

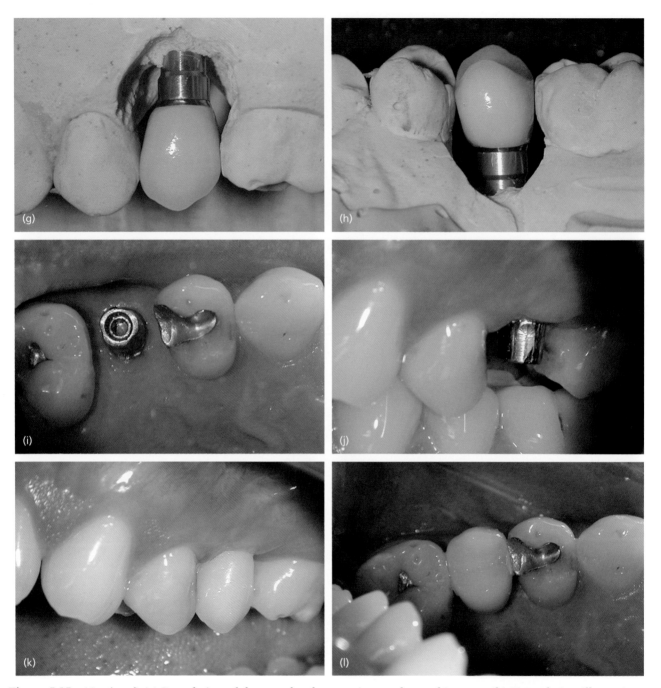

Figure 5.15 (*Continued*) (g) Buccal view of the completed restoration on the working cast. (h) Lingual view illustrating the emergence profile. (i, j) Abutment in place: (i) clinical view and (j) buccal view. (k) Porcelain fused to the seated metal restoration. (l) Occlusal view of the completed restoration in place.

completed restoration can be looked at on the working cast to consider the emergence profile.

The abutment is then placed in situ and an electronic driver used to torque to the recommended value. Porcelain can then be fused to the metal restoration. This author typically uses an electronic torque driver to tighten the screw, waiting a short time and reapplying the tightening torque once again. The restoration can be placed with a temporary cement (Temp Bond™) for a period of a few week or months to be certain that no adjustments are necessary and then

cemented with a more permanent cement. The contours of the final restoration should replicate those of the adjacent natural bicuspid.

Nobel Biocare Unaltered Abutments: Two Teeth Replacement

The procedure for placing more than one implant with prefabricated Nobel Biocare abutments is shown in Figure 5.16. A prefabricated Easy Abutment comes packaged with an abutment screw, impression syringe

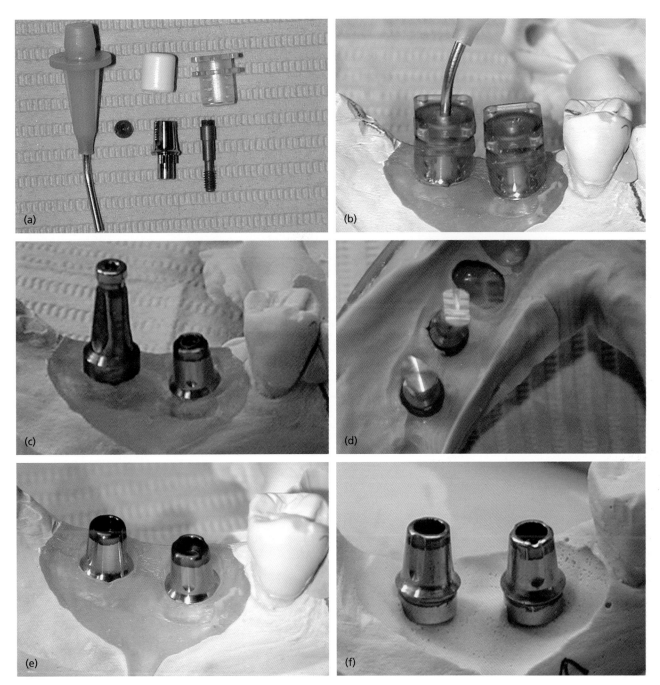

Figure 5.16 (a) Components of a prefabricated Easy Abutment set. (b) Making the implant impression. (c) Impression coping for an implant-level impression (left) and Easy Abutment (right). (d) Implant-level analogs in place in the impression prior to pouring with die stone. (e) Resulting working cast with the two abutments in place. Wide diameter implants (5 mm) were placed to replace the missing first and second molars. (f) Working cast with soft tissue-replicating material removed for optimal access to the margin areas. Note the indexing grooves on the abutments.

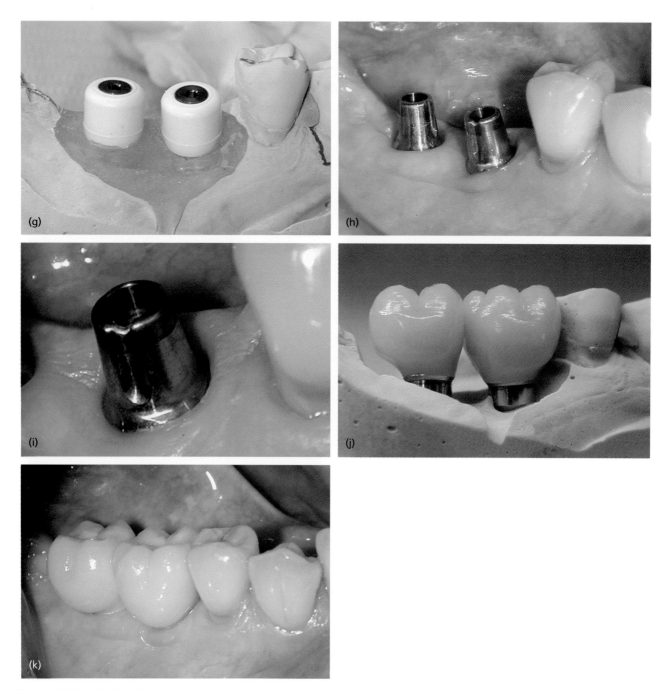

Figure 5.16 (*Continued*) (g) Abutment temporary caps on the working cast. (h) Clinical view of the abutments in place. (i) Close-up of the soft tissue–abutment relationship. (j) Completed restorations on the working cast. Note the smooth emergence profile and gradual increase in crown diameter. (k) Cemented restorations in place.

tip, impression snap cap, screw access hole seal, and temporary cap.

Once the abutments are placed, plastic impression caps are placed over them and snapped on to the beveled edge. The syringe tip is attached to the impression injection gun and material expressed into the snap cap through the occlusal hole. The tray is filled and the impression completed. If the abutment is placed in the mouth, the snap cap can be positioned and an analog can be used in the working cast to construct the restoration. If any modifications to the abutment are required it is best to take implant-level impressions. Once the implant-level analogs are in place in the impression, prior to pouring with die stone, it is always sensible to rinse the impression and remove any debris. Then gently dry the recess with air prior to placing the analog/impression coping in the impression. Use a high-quality, low-expansion die stone to pour the master cast. Soft tissue-replicating material is then placed around the analogs.

Indexing grooves should be made on the abutments. If modifications are made to the abutments, additional markings will need to be applied to avoid seating confusion. Temporary caps are placed over the abutments on the working cast. The cap surfaces are smooth and the centrally located small retention screw keeps the cap firmly in place clinically. Ideal implant spacing is required to prevent contact between adjacent caps. In the event there is a proximal space issue, the sides can be shaved down with a rotary diamond instrument and polished.

The abutments are then clinically placed. These abutments work exceptionally well when there is ideal spacing and axial orientation of the implants. If major modifications are necessary, the retention integrity of the walls may be compromised. It is important to achieve the correct relationship between the soft tissue and abutment. A near 45-degree shoulder bevel allows adequate room for an optimal porcelain–metal interface and a smooth esthetic emergence profile.

The restorations are completed on the working cast and then cemented in place. Unmodified and minimally modified abutments offer good crown retention. Temporary cementation is recommended. This author's preference is Temp Bond cement as it provides good long-term retention and the crowns, if necessary, can be retrieved without damage.

Implant Direct Straight Contoured Abutment

The procedure for the placement of an Implant Direct RePlant™ straight contoured abutment is shown in Figure 5.17.

If the contoured shoulder is above the tissue level it will need modification. The gingival/occlusal length may also require alteration. As the contoured shoulder is modified and brought lower to the tissue level, the shoulder width reduces but the near-parallel wall integrity is maintained.

To match the round 4.3 mm diameter of the implant loading table, prefabricated abutments have a typically rounded shape. The cervical shape of the clinical crown of a bicuspid, however, is ovoid in shape. That creates a contour discrepancy that can be seen in the proximal view of this example. These limitations can only be overcome by the use of a custom milled or cast abutment.

In modifying the cervical collar in the restoration shown in Figure 5.17, the buccal aspect was contoured lower than the lingual to insure that the metal collar did not show clinically. Once the restoration modification is finished, it can be cemented in place. The restoration should match the natural contours of the occlusal table and contact areas.

Esthetic results can be obtained with prefabricated abutments. More often than not, however, modifications have to be made in order to achieve an optimal result.

Implant Direct Prefabricated Abutment Modification

The procedure for the placement and modification of an Implant Direct RePlant prefabricated abutment is shown in Figure 5.18. In this example there are three implants replacing the maxillary right first molar, a bicuspid, and and a cuspid. Tissue depth measurements were made on the cast prior to ordering the abutments. This insures that the appropriate cervical collar height is selected.

Changes can then be made to the abutments. Note that sufficient metal bulk is needed to permit modifications. Alterations can also include dropping the abutment and reducing and re-contouring the facial aspects of the abutments. In this example, efforts were made to bring the body of the abutment into the center axis of the crown. On the working cast, the shoulder margins were below the soft tissue and the prep walls were still very parallel.

The abutments can then be placed clinically. The screw access holes can be blocked out by condensing Teflon tape and sealed with Cavit.

The completed crowns are first examined on the working cast. Custom milled or cast abutments can have a more accurate emergence profile. In this clinical case, the papillae between the cuspid and the lateral were preserved. It is more difficult to preserve papillae with round abutments.

The final emergence profile of a crown with a round prefabricated abutment (Figure 5.19a) does not exactly replicate the natural contours of the tooth. The natural

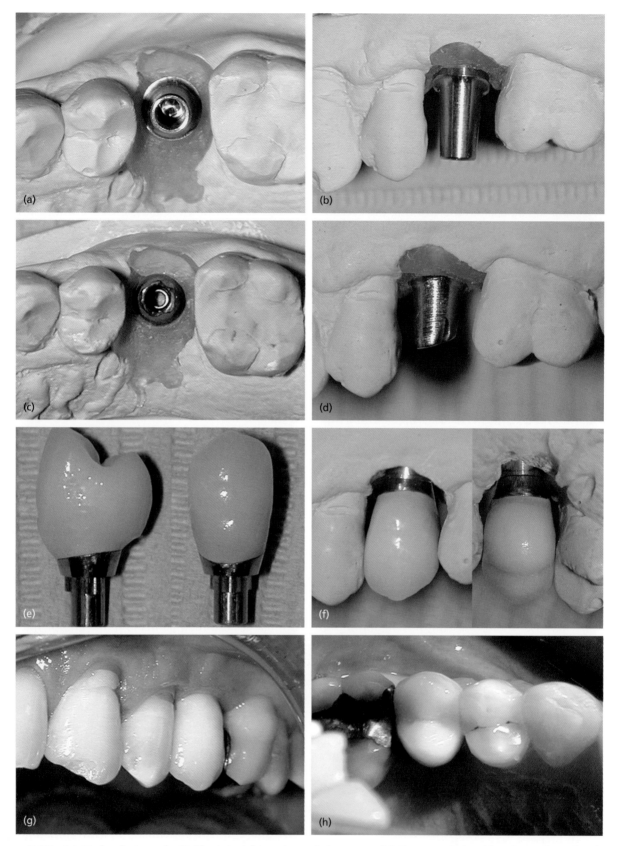

Figure 5.17 (a) Occlusal view of a RePlant straight contoured abutment. (b) Contoured shoulder above tissue level and the gingival/occlusal length, both needing modification. (c) Occlusal view of the modified abutment. (d) Facial view illustrating the modified shoulder height and width. A small facial indexing notch is present on the distofacial side for orientation. (e, f) Completed metal-ceramic restoration: (e) facial (left) and proximal (right) views, and (f) buccal (left) and lingual (right) views. (g) Facial view of the cemented restoration in situ. The adjacent bicuspid is slightly rotated towards the distal, making the restoration on no. 13 appear to be slightly wider. A healthy band of attached tissue is also present. (h) Occlusal view of the restoration illustrating the natural contours of the occlusal table and contact areas.

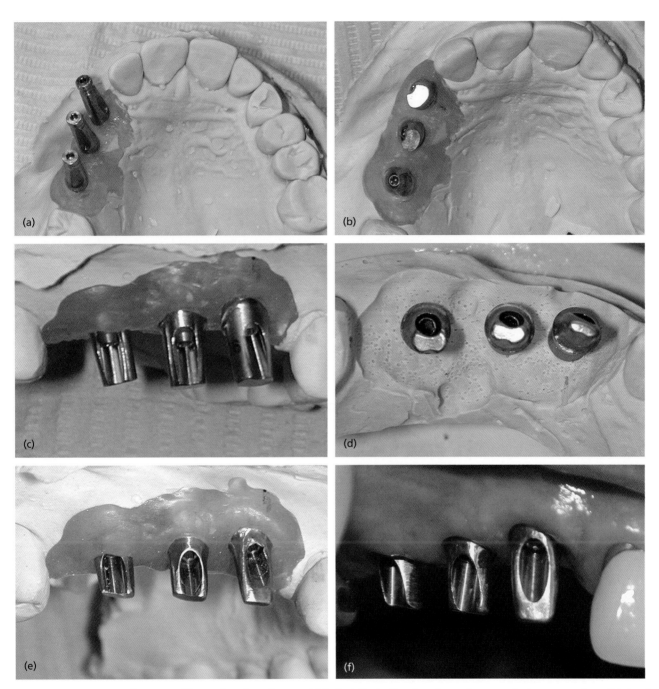

Figure 5.18 (a) Working cast illustrating that the cuspid is facially inclined and requires angulation correction. (b) Angle abutment in the no. 6 location and straight prefab abutments on the remaining two implants. (c) Facial view of the abutments prior to modification being made. The shoulder on the cuspid abutment was dropped apically a couple of millimeters. (d, e) Completed re-contoured abutments on the working cast: (d) occlusal view and (e) facial view. (f) Abutments in place clinically.

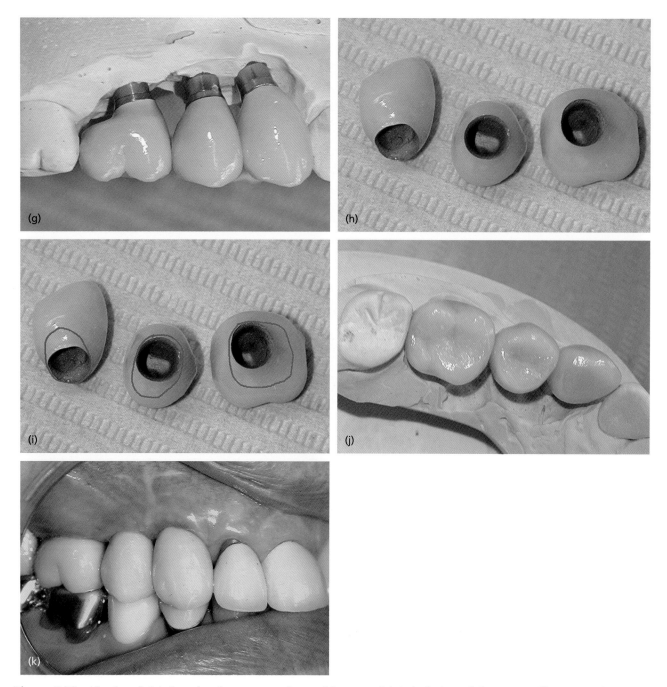

Figure 5.18 (*Continued*) (g) Completed crowns on the working cast. (h) Apical view of the crowns illustrating the size discrepancy of the crown to abutment and of the circular abutments' loading platform. (i) Red line indicating the more ideal shape of a custom milled or cast abutment. (j) Occlusal view of the completed restorations showing the effort to reduce the occlusal table. (k) Facial view of the completed restorations in situ.

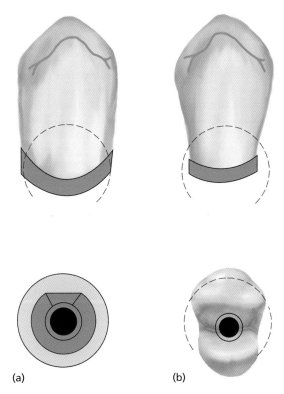

Figure 5.19 (a) Typical contour generated with a round prefabricated abutment. (b) Tapering down of the crown contour (waist).

tooth typically has a waist that is narrower at the proximal. The tapering down of the crown contour (waist) is illustrated in Figure 5.19b. The faciolingual contour is also much more elongated and tapered towards the lingual. These dimensional changes are difficult to overcome with round or slightly flared prefabricated abutments.

REFERENCES AND ADDITIONAL READING

Andersson, B., Glauser, R., Maglione, M., & Taylor, A. (2003) Ceramic implant abutments for short-span FPDs: a prospective 5 year multicenter study. *International Journal of Prosthodontics*, 16, 640–647.

Andersson, B., Taylor, A., Lang, B.R., et al. (2001). Alumina ceramic implant abutments uses for single tooth replacement: a prospective 1 to 3 year multicenter study. *International Journal of Prosthodontics*, 14, 432–438.

Barbarosa, G.A., Simamoto Junior P.C., Fernandes Neto, A.J., de Mattos Mda G., Neves, F. D. (2007). Prosthetic laboratory influence on the vertical misfit at the implant/UCLA abutment interface. *Brazilian Dental Journal*, 18(2), 139–43.

Byrne, D., Houston, F., Cleary, R., & Claffey, N. (1998). The fit of cast and premachined implant abutments. *Journal of Prosthetic Dentistry*, 80, 184–92.

Chandra, S., Chandra, S., Chandra, S. (2008). *Textbook of Dental and Oral Anatomy, Physiology and Occlusion*. New Delhi: Jaypee Brothers Medical Publishers.

Drago, C.J. (1991). Partially edentulous prosthodontic reconstruction using the Branemark implant system. In *Dental Implant Prosthodontics*, ed. Caswell, C.W. & Clark, A.E. Philadelphia: JB Lippencott, 59–91.

Geurs, N.C., Vassilopoulos, P.J., & Reddy, M.S. (2011). Histologic evidence of connective tissue integration on laser microgrooved abutments in humans. *Clinical Advances in Periodontics*, 1, 29–33.

Glauser, R., Sailer, I., Wohlwend, A., Studer, S., Schibli, M., & Scharer, P. (2004). Experimental zirconia abutments for implant supported single-tooth restorations in esthetically demanding regions: 4-year results of a prospective clinical study. *International Journal of Prosthodontics*, 17, 285–290.

Heydecke, G., Sierraalta, M., (2002). Razzoog, M.E. Evolution and use of aluminum oxide single-tooth implant abutments: a short review and presentation of two cases. *International Journal of Prosthodontics*, 15, 488–493.

Jemt, T. (1986). Modified single and short span restorations supported by osseointegrated fixtures in the partially edentulous jaw. *Journal of Prosthetic Dentistry*, 55, 243–246.

Kan, J.Y.K., Rungcharassaeng, K., Bohsali, K., Goodacre, C.J., & Lang, B.R. (1999). Clinical methods for evaluating implant framework fit. *Journal of Prosthetic Dentistry*, 81, 7–13.

Krogh, P.H.J. (1986). Site selection for the placement of osseointegrated implants in the totally edentulous maxilla and the partially edentulous mandible and maxilla. In *Tissue Integration in Oral and Maxillofacial Reconstruction*, ed. VanSteenburge, D. Amsterdam: Excerpta Medica, 344–346.

Kucey, B.K.S. & Fraser, D.C. (2000). The Procera abutment: the fifth generation abutment for dental implants. *Journal of the Canadian Dental Association*, 66, 445.

Lewis, S., Beumer, J., III, Hornburg, W., & Moy, P. (1988). The "UCLA" abutment. *International Journal of Oral and Maxillofacial Implants*, 3, 183–9.

Lewis, S.G., Liamas, D., & Avera, S. (1992). The UCLA abutment: a four-year review. *Journal of Prosthetic Dentistry*, 67, 509–515.

Nevins, M., Camelo, M., Nevins, M.L., Schupbach, P., Kim, D.M. (2012) Connective Tissue Attachment to Laser-Microgrooved Abutments: A Human Histologic Case Report. *International Journal of Periodontics and Restorative Dentistry* 32:385–392.

Nevins, M., Camelo, M., Nevins, M.L., Schupbach, P., Kim, D.M. (2012) Reattachment of Connective Tissue Fibers to a Laser-Microgrooved Abutment Surface. *International Journal of Periodontics and Restorative Dentistry* 32:e131–e134.

Nevins, M., Kim, D.M., Jun, S.H., Guze, K., Schupbach, P., & Nevins, M.L. (2010). Histologic evidence of a connective tissue attachment to laser microgrooved abutments: a canine study. *International Journal of Periodontics and Restorative Dentistry*, 30, 245–255.

Nevins, M., Nevins, M.L., Camelo, M., Boyesen, J.L., & Kim, D.M. (2008). Human histologic evidence of a connective tissue attachment to a dental implant. *International Journal of Periodontics and Restorative Dentistry*, 28, 111–121.

Niznick, G. & Misch, C.E. (1988). The Core-Vent system of osseointegrated implants. In *Clinical Dentistry*, Vol. 5, ed. Clark, J.W. & Harden, J.F. Philadelphia: JB Lippencott, 1–11.

Pecora, G.E., Ceccarelli, R., Bonelli, M., Alexander, H., & Ricci, J.L. (2009). Clinical evaluation of laser microtexturing for soft tissue and bone attachment to dental implants. *Implant Dentistry*, 18, 57–66.

Piconi, C., & Maccauro, G. (1999). Zirconia as a ceramic biomaterial. *Biomaterials*, 20, 1.

Presipino, V. & Ingber, A. (1993). Esthetic high strength implant abutments part 1. *Journal of Esthetic Dentistry*, 5, 29–36.

Silveira, C.D., Jr, Fernandes Neto, A.J., Neves, F.D., Franco, S.D., & Mendonca, G. (2002). Laboratory procedures influence in the implant/UCLA abutment fit – pilot study. *Brazilian Dental Journal* 4, 392–400.

Sullivan, D.T. (1986). Prosthetic considerations for the utilization of osseointegrated fixtures in the partially edentulous arch. *International Journal of Oral and Maxillofacial Implants*, 1, 39–45.

Watkin, A. & Kerstein, R.B. (2008). Improving darkened anterior peri-implant tissue color with zirconia custom implant abutments. *Compendium of Continuing Education in Dentistry*, 29(4), 238–240, 242.

6

Use of CAD/CAM Technology in Custom Abutment Manufacturing

Julian Osorio¹ and Robert B. Kerstein²

¹Department of Restorative Dentistry, Division of Graduate and Post Graduate Prosthodontics, Tufts University School of Dental Medicine, Boston, MA
²Private Practice, Boston, MA

HISTORY OF CAD/CAM TECHNOLOGY IN PROSTHETIC DENTISTRY

Computer-aided design (CAD)/computer-aided milling (CAM) technology first appeared in prosthetic dentistry with the introduction of the first CEREC scanning and milling system in 1985 (Siemens AG, Germany) (Calamia 1994; Isenberg and Garber 1994). CEREC is an acronym for "chairside economical restoration of esthetic ceramics." The first CEREC system photographed the cavity preparation and stored the photograph as a 3-dimensional (3D) digital model. Next, the proprietary software approximated the restoration shape using biogeneric comparisons with the surrounding teeth. The clinician could then refine that model using 3D CAD software, after which an optical scanner controlled a milling machine that carved the actual restoration out of a ceramic block using diamond head cutters. The milled ceramic restoration was then bonded into the tooth using a resin cement.

Another early CAD/CAM system was the CELAY system (Mikrona Technologie AG, Switzerland) (Eidenbenz et al. 1994; McLaren and Sorensen 1994). The CELAY system had some advantages over the early CEREC system as it could create all surfaces of a restoration, whereas the earliest CEREC system could not fabricate the occlusal surface. Another advantage was that the CELAY system had the potential to fabricate crowns and short-span bridges utilizing the In-Ceram system (Vita Zahnfabrik, Bad Säckingen, Switzerland) (Eidenbenz et al. 1994). Both the CEREC and CELAY systems could be used for direct and indirect restoration fabrication so the clinician could opt for completing a milled ceramic restoration in a single patient appointment. This is still an attribute of the current day CEREC 3D system.

Through most of the 1980s and 1990s, CEREC outpaced CELAY with production advances and became the predominant CAD/CAM chairside milling system in clinical use. Both its software and milling hardware have undergone numerous changes and CEREC can now offer clinicians sophisticated ideal tooth morphology design and milling capability. A second generation scanning and milling unit was developed in 1994, which was followed 8 years later in 2002 by the CEREC 3D system (the first Windows®-based CEREC product) (Figure 6.1).

The CEREC technology spawned an entire speciality of prosthetic dentistry that, at present, comprises over 100 milling systems that produce implant abutments, copings, removable partial denture frameworks, fixed

Clinical and Laboratory Manual of Dental Implant Abutments, First Edition. Edited by Hamid R. Shafie.
© 2014 John Wiley & Sons, Inc. Published 2014 by John Wiley & Sons, Inc.

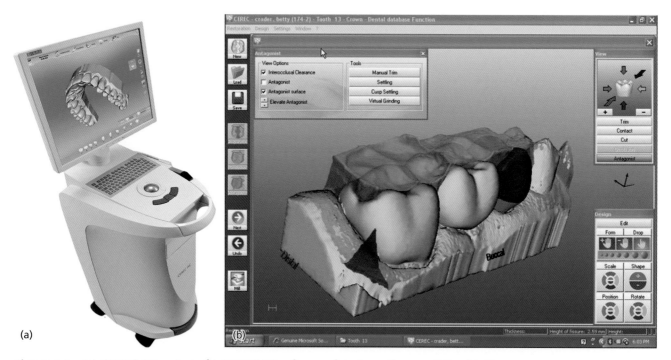

Figure 6.1   (a) CEREC 3D system. (b) CEREC 3D software planning a three-unit fixed bridge.

bridge frameworks, fixed implant frameworks, crowns, inlays, onlays, and porcelain veneers.

HISTORY OF CAD/CAM TECHNOLOGY IN IMPLANT ABUTMENT MANUFACTURING

CAD/CAM custom manufacturing technology developed at a time when custom abutment options for implants were mostly created manually by technicians utilizing a UCLA wax-up sleeve (Branemark Implants, Gothenberg, Sweden) that fitted over an external hex platform design (Nishimura et al. 1999). The UCLA plastic sleeve acted as scaffold to hold a technician-created wax-up that shaped the custom abutment form. The wax-up was invested with the abutment connection, so that after burn-out, cast gold formed the abutment, which was mechanically adhered to the connection. The abutment then screwed over an external hex onto the implant body. Later UCLA plastic designs incorporated the external hex into the plastic waxing sleeve so that the entire waxed abutment was a one-piece abutment. This could then be secured onto the hex with an abutment screw.

Adaptations to the UCLA design came from other implant manufacturers (e.g. Core-Vent, Van Nuys, CA, USA), who created preformed plastic waxing compo-

nents that fitted inside the implant. These plastic burn-out components could be trimmed and waxed onto so as to form ideal tooth preparation forms that, after casting in gold, would fit back into the implant body. The cast abutments were internally cemented to the implant instead of being screwed into place like the traditional UCLA abutment. Recurrent clinical problems were observed with these internally cemented, castable abutments. One was dislodgement due to problems with the cementation. Another was fracture of the internally cemented post (which rendered the internal compartment of the implant body useless). Such problems resulted in cementable abutments losing clinical acceptance to the internally hexed, screw-retained custom abutments.

The first manufactured CAD/CAM abutment technology utilized in implant–abutment prosthodontics was described in 2000 as the Atlantis Custom Abutment Technology (Atlantis Components, Cambridge, MA, USA) (Figure 6.2) (Kerstein et al. 2000). Osorio, in collaboration with Atlantis Components, secured the first patents on computer-aided *virtual design technology* for implant abutments (Osorio 1997; Osorio et al. 1999, 2001).

The earliest Atlantis abutment design capability eliminated the need for a technician-created wax-up by employing design software that contained numerous virtual tools to create the abutment virtually (VAD™, Atlantis Components). First, a master cast was

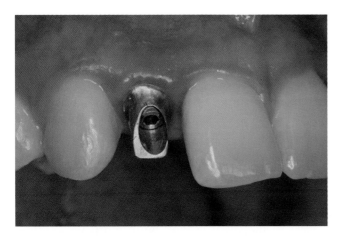

Figure 6.2 Early Atlantis abutment in the no. 7 site.

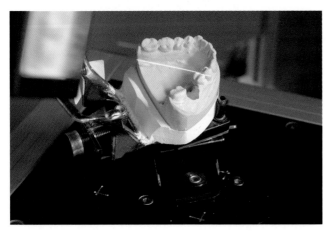

Figure 6.3 Optical scanning of a master cast.

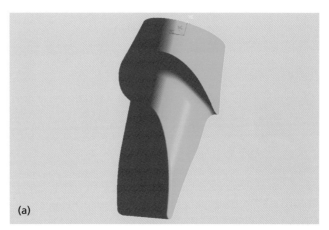

(a)

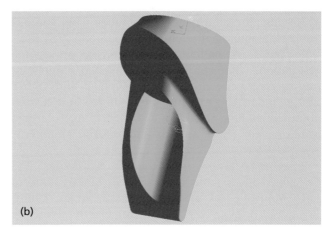

(b)

Figure 6.4 (a) Earliest virtual incisor design template. (b) Earliest virtual abutment file type that was exported for milling the abutment shown in (a).

made from an intra-oral transfer impression that located: (i) the intra-arch position of the implant to be restored; (ii) the soft tissue contours around the implant; (iii) the neighboring teeth; and (iv) the opposing occlusal clearance. This master cast and its opposing cast were scanned individually (Figure 6.3), and then virtually articulated within the design software.

The virtual abutment design templates of the incisors (Figure 6.4a), canines, premolars, and molars could then be modified using numerous measurement and design tools, to create a virtual *patient-specific* abutment (Figure 6.4b).

When the virtual design was complete, the digital abutment files were exported to a milling machine where commercially available pure titanium blanks were milled into the final abutment (see Figure 6.2). The milling of the blanks included: (i) the abutment screw access; (ii) differing abutment connections to accommodate many different implant systems; (iii) the

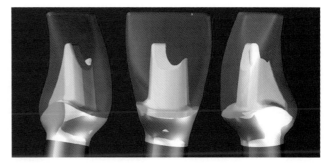

Figure 6.5 Three virtual design views of an early central incisor Atlantis custom abutment.

hex (either internal or external); (iv) the cuspal contours and occlusal morphology; (v) a shoulder or chamfer margin; and (vi) the abutment base, which was shaped to maximize an ideal tooth preparation form despite screw access (Figure 6.5).

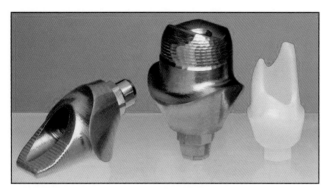

Figure 6.6   Atlantis gold hue, titanium, and zirconia custom abutments (left to right).

Because the abutments were milled from computer files, a single abutment could be duplicated multiple times. A patient could wear a provisional restoration, while the lab technician had a duplicate one to create the final crown (Kerstein and Osorio 2003). Today, the Atlantis virtual design and custom abutment milling technology is used to manufacture titanium, gold hue, and zirconia custom abutments (Figure 6.6).

Prior to Atlantis, the Procera® technology was developed in the mid-1990s (Nobel Biocare Procera LLC, Mahwah, NJ, USA) (Andersson et al. 1998). Procera technology was initially capable of fabricating all-ceramic crowns. Later, the Procera system expanded to include the fabrication of custom abutments. These abutments were initially formed from a technician-created wax-up made on a plastic waxing sleeve that inserted into an implant analog. When the wax-up was complete, it was scanned and then milled out of blocks of ceramic materials. Today, the wax-up sleeve is still required to create Procera abutments. However, after being manually inserted into an implant analog, the wax-up sleeve and master cast are scanned into design software so that the abutment shape can be then virtually waxed-up.

The most notable differences between the early Atlantis abutment and the Procera abutment manufacturing processes were:

- The Procera abutment contours were the result of a technician's waxed-up morphology.
- The Procera milled abutment was (and still is today) attached to the implant via a *metal connecting element* that is screwed through when inserting the abutment into the implant. This separate metallic connection incorporates an additional location within the implant–abutment system where the solidity of the screw anchorage can be compromised under occlusal function. This can result in increased risk of abutment dislodgements and zirconia fractures.

- The Procera system is a "closed system" that can only be utilized with Nobel Biocare implants (Nobel Biocare LLC, Yorba Linda, CA, USA).
- Atlantis titanium abutments did not rely on a technician-created wax-up for abutment contour.
- Atlantis titanium abutments did not require a separate metallic connection component to engage the implant. This was because they were virtually designed and milled from the implant connection all the way up to the cuspal contours. The connection to the implant was milled in one piece in titanium without additional locations within the implant–abutment system where the solidity of the screw anchorage could be compromised under occlusal function. This is still the case today for titanium and zirconia Atlantis abutments.
- Atlantis technology is not a "closed system." It can be employed with over 50 different implant connections, including the connections from but not limited to Astratech (Astratech/Atlantis, Waltham, MA, USA), Nobel Biocare (Nobel Biocare LLC), Biomet 3i (Biomet 3i, Palm Beach Gardens, FL, USA), Zimmer (Zimmer Dental, Carlsbad, CA, USA), Straumann (Straumann USA LLC, Andover, MA, USA), Dentsply/Friadent (Friadent GmbH, Manheim, Germany), and BioHorizons (BioHorizons, Birmingham, AL, USA). The Atlantis VAD software incorporates the connection size and shape parameters of various implants, and mills the custom abutment for these different connection designs. This flexibility allows the restorative dentist to use a single custom abutment system even if his/her surgical team utilizes many different types of implants.

The next early CAD/CAM abutment system was the Encode System™ (Biomet 3i) (Drago and Peterson 2007). The Encode System scanned a cast made from an intra-oral impression that measured the position of different-sized healing caps that contained orientating surface lines. The different-sized healing caps fit specific underlying implant sizes, and the surface orientating lines predicted the rotational position of the underlying implant. From these combinations of scanned measurements, in combination with a technician-created wax-up, the Encode software could create a custom abutment for the underlying implant, which was milled for intra-oral use. Encode is available today as a closed system and can only be used with 3i implants.

This chapter will discuss the Atlantis patient-specific custom abutment manufacturing technology, which spawned the entire custom abutment manufacturing segment of implant prosthodontics. At present, most other major implant companies have developed their own custom abutment manufacturing processes. However, these alternative systems follow the original Procera model by employing a *wax–scan–mill* approach that is technician driven and not software driven. Only the Atlantis process completely creates the abutment within a virtual environment before it is manufactured.

Table 6.1 describes some of the advantages and disadvantages of a number of commercially available manufactured custom abutment solutions.

VIRTUAL DESIGN AND MANUFACTURE OF ABUTMENTS

Design Process Prior to Machining Custom Abutments

The Atlantis custom abutment manufacturing process, which utilizes virtual abutment design software (Atlantis VAD, Astratech/Atlantis,Waltham, MA, USA), is an ISO 13485 certified and Food and Drug Administration (FDA) Quality System Regulation (QSR) compliant process. A manufactured custom abutment is first virtually created within the design software by *virtual tools* before it is machine milled. Before the virtual design process can start, a *non-virtual* implant master cast must be fabricated. The master cast contains all the implant analogs (that reproduce the intra-oral implant placements) surrounded by a removable soft tissue reproduction. Soft tissue removability allows for fit and placement evaluations of the final custom abutments; the abutment bases are fabricated anatomically wider than the implant body and the intra-oral peri-implant sulci.

Laboratory Steps in the Scanning and Fabrication of Custom Abutments

The steps in the scanning and fabrication of a custom abutment are shown in Figure 6.7. Master cast fabrication begins with the intra-oral placement of all the impression copings.

After radiographic confirmation that the impression copings are properly seated, the master impression can be made with an elastomeric impression material (Impregum, 3M Espe, Seefeld, Germany). The recovered impression is cleaned of blood and saliva, and then disinfected appropriately. The impression copings are removed from each implant, and the matched analogs placed onto each impression coping. They inserted back into their respective location within the impression guided by the individual copings' axial wall shape.

Once all the impression copings are in place, the peri-implant tissues can be reproduced within the impression. A soft denture reline material (Zhermack Occludefast, River Edge, NJ, USA) is mixed and spatulated around the analogs. The occlusal third of the analog body is covered with the soft tissue material, leaving the apical two-thirds exposed. This allows the analog's retentive elements to engage the die stone when it is poured. When the soft tissue is completely set, it is trimmed with a blade into a block-like shape that facilitates its easy removal and accurate replacement back into the final master cast. The removal and replacement of the soft tissue is crucial for the technician to be able to evaluate the seating of any oversized and fully anatomically designed abutments.

The die stone pour is accomplished in two stages. First, the impression is held inverted and vacuum-mixed die stone (Fuji Rock EP, GC America, Alsip, IL, USA) is vibrated into the impression. This is done until the intaglio surface and the retentive elements of each analog are completely covered with stone. Then, a rubber model base former is filled, after which the first pour is inverted onto the former so both pours together set completely.

The master cast is retrieved, trimmed, articulated, and smoothed externally. Because of the block cut of the soft tissue made prior to the die stone pour, the entire soft tissue element can be removed to simplify the seating of any oversized and fully anatomical abutments.

The master cast is then ready for optical scanning to begin the virtual abutment design.

Virtual Abutment Design of Custom Abutments

The sequence of steps involved in virtual abutment design can be seen in Figure 6.8. The procedure shows a mandibular right posterior quadrant that is to be restored with a single PFM crown (tooth no. 28) and two implant-supported splinted crowns in the no. 29 and no. 30 sites.

The stone master cast and its opposing cast are scanned and imported into the design software where they are reassembled and virtually occluded. Note in Figure 6.8d that there are two "holes" within the edentulous area where the implants have been "located" within the scanned cast. To facilitate ease of cast viewing during the design process, the occluded casts can be virtually rotated 360 degrees within the design software.

Next, virtual crowns are placed upon each implant (and any neighboring teeth that are being restored as well) and properly stretched into opposing occlusal contact. They are then virtually contoured to match the anatomic requirements of the neighboring teeth. In Figure 6.8e tooth no. 28 is virtually crowned in a pink-colored translucent restoration (denoting the presence of a neighboring non-implant restoration),

Table 6.1 Comparison Chart of Some of the Commercially Available Custom Abutment Systems

	Astra Tech Atlantis™ Abutment	Nobel Biocare Procera®	Straumann Etkon	Biomet 3i Encode®	Zimmer Dental Patient-specific abutments	Whip Mix Vericore®	Glidewell Inclusive® Implant Abutment	GC Aadva™ Abutments
Interfaces	Over 50 interfaces, including Astra Tech, Nobel Biocare, Straumann, Biomet 3i, Zimmer Dental, BioHorizons, Keystone Dental, Sybron Dental Solutions	NobelReplace®, NobelActive®, Branemark, Strauman RN, Astra Tech (titanium only)	Straumann only	Biomet 3i only	Zimmer only	29 including Astra Tech, Biomet 3i, Nobel Biocare, Straumann, Zimmer Dental	NobelReplace, Biomet 3i Certain®, Zimmer Screw-Vent®, NobelActive, Branemark RP, Straumann Bone Level, Neoss	Nobel Biocare, Biomet 3i, Straumann, Astra Tech, Sybron Dental Solutions
Materials								
Titanium	X	X	X	X	X		X	X
Gold-shaded titanium	X			X				
Zirconia, white	X	X	X	X	X	X	X	X
Zirconia, shaded	X	X				X		
Advantages	Only "intelligent" system with computer-assisted built-in design parameters. Eliminates manual wax-up aspects of abutment design. Can be employed with both simple and complex cases. Engineered abutments insures precision. Computer files can be used many times; allows for duplicate abutments and later orders. Compatible with all major implant systems. Comprehensive range of material options	Is a solution for removable prostheses like bar overdentures	Broad range of crown and bridge options (Ti, Zr, CrCo; burn-out resin and an acrylic option for provisional restorations)	Impression of implant can be made without removing healing abutment	Precise friction fit	Open architecture-accepting shape can fabricate copings and bridge frameworks. Zirconia abutments in 8 shades and 31 platform options. Custom-milled titanium overdenture bars	Multiple interface options	Can fabricate copings, bridges, and abutments in multiple zirconia shades. Compatible with all major implant systems
Disadvantages	• No manual abutment design alterations possible	• Design software is difficult to use • Product often does not match request	• Turnaround times can be lengthy even for titanium • Requires purchase of scanner • Closed system • Small number of scanning labs	• Available to trained and skilled designers • Robotic analog placement has been shown to be inaccurate • Closed system	• Fairly long turnaround times • Closed system • No gold-shaded option	• No titanium abutments • Limited control of abutment and bar design for non-scanning labs	• Lack of design control due to rrquired wax up • No documentation or research on process predictability • Long turnaround times	• No gold-shaded option • Abutments not engineered

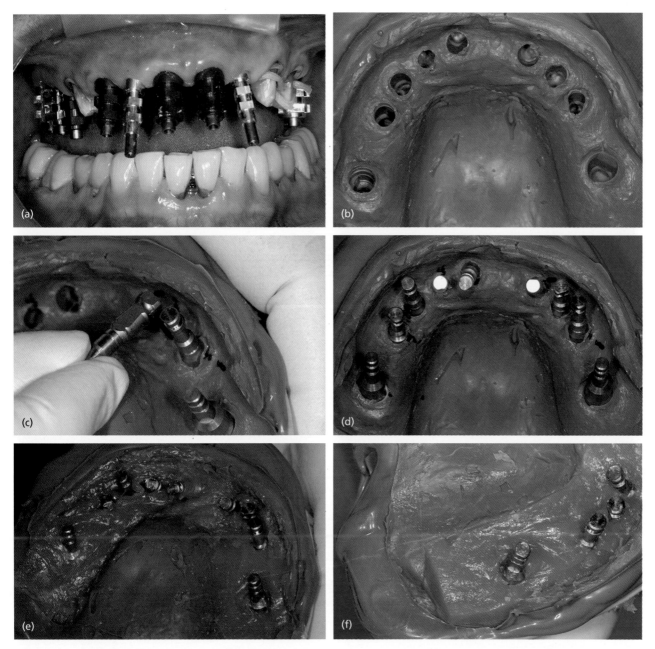

Figure 6.7 (a) Intra-oral placement of impression copings. (b) Master impression. (c) Matched implant analogs are placed onto each impression coping, and inserted back into their respective location within the impression. (d) All the analogs inserted into the master Impression. (e) Soft denture reline material around the analogs. (f) After setting, the soft tissue is trimmed into a block-like shape.

while the implant virtual crowns in the no. 29 and no. 30 sites are represented in translucent green.

These virtual crown shapes will guide the future form of the underlying abutment to be designed in the same manner that a full contour wax-up and clear plastic template overlay would guide the manual creation of a cast custom abutment. The design software allows for easy removal (and replacement) of the

implants, virtual crowns, and opposing cast so that all the case elements can be viewed with varying transparencies. Virtual crowns can also be displayed as a meshwork should the abutment designer prefers this to a transparent view.

All these desktop display features enhance the designer's ability to visualize all anatomic aspects of the case. Under these optimally shaped virtual crowns,

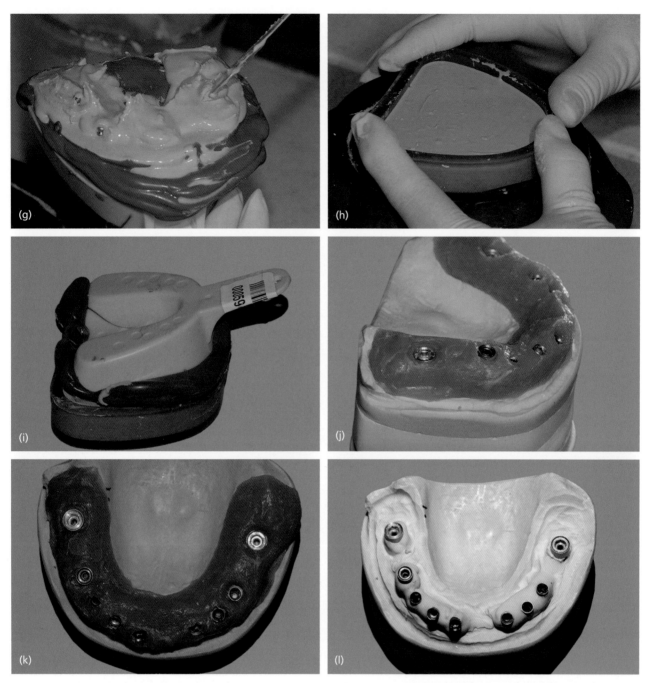

Figure 6.7 (*Continued*) (g) The first stone pour. (h) The second stone pour. (i) The first pour is inverted onto the model base former so both pours set together. (j, k) Master cast trimmed, articulated, and smoothed externally: (j) lateral view and (k) occlusal view. (l) Completed master cast with the soft tissue reproduction removed.

the ideal abutment morphology is generated from the external crown contours. The abutment morphology is therefore designed to properly fit underneath the individual final restoration. Figure 6.8g shows the implant angulations being corrected with the ideal abutment morphology within the virtual cast, in the same way that the final abutments will sit intra-orally to facilitate ideal restoration of the patient's edentulous region.

Once the ideal abutment morphology has been virtually designed, the digital files are exported to the milling machinery for the manufacture of the final abutments. In this example, note how both abutments follow the opposing occlusal plane for future final crown fabrication. The final abutment form is a definitive match to the virtually designed abutments and will support the crown morphology that was also virtually designed.

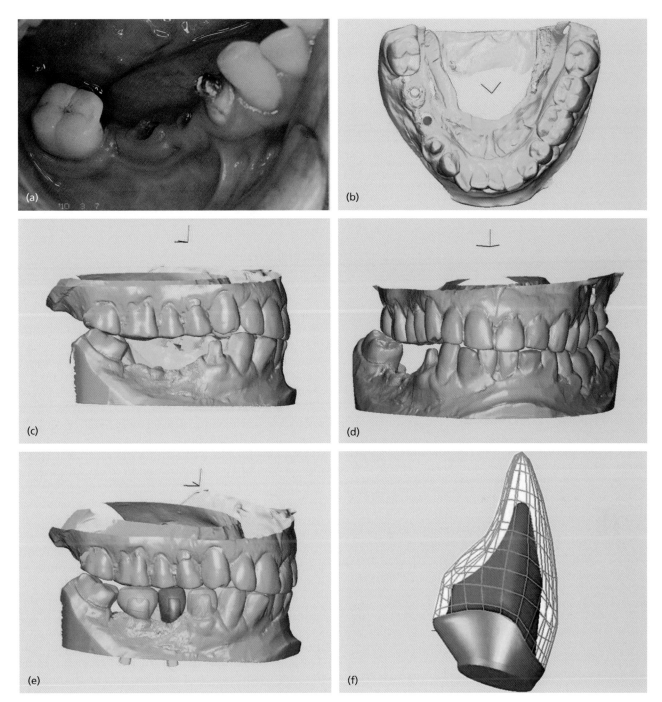

Figure 6.8 (a) Edentulous ridge with implants and prepared tooth no. 28. (b) Scanned master cast of tooth no. 28. (c, d) Different views of the virtually occluded master cast and opposing cast. (e) Virtual crowns over teeth nos 28, 29, and 30. (f) Virtual crown meshwork.

Machine Milling of Custom Abutments

Although custom abutments began as traditional cast gold abutments, today the most frequent materials to be used are titanium, zirconium dioxide, and plastic (for provisional abutments). Custom abutments are milled from titanium or ceramic rods once the virtual design of the abutment is completed. The digital abutment files guide the cutting tools of the milling machines in 6 degrees of freedom through the differing abutment material(s) to manufacture a finished custom abutment.

Milling machines range in size, rate of abutment production, and cutting degrees of freedom. A typical

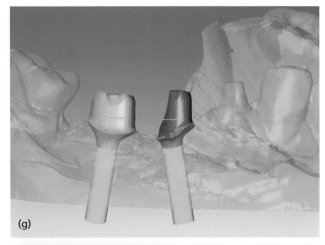

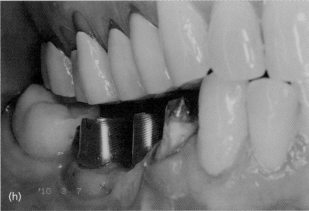

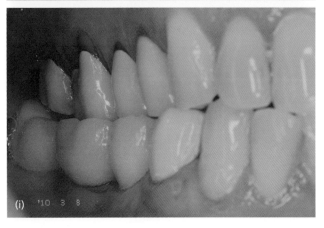

Figure 6.8 (*Continued*) (g) Virtual correction of the alignment of poorly angled implants. (h) Abutments in place with opposing occlusion. (i) Restoration in place.

milling machine can be seen in Figure 6.9. This machine mills long rods of commercially pure titanium within its milling chamber (rod materials milled are FDA 510K cleared) (Figure 6.10). Approximately 12 different abutments can be cut out of each foot-length of a titanium rod.

The milling takes place under copious amounts of cooling water spray (Figure 6.11).

When milling tools require replacement due to production wear, the milling machine self-manages the automated tool replacement. Depending on the product to be milled, the individual machines have their own "self-check" system in place, which monitors preprogrammed machining parameters while the milling process continually produces abutments. When the cutting tools fail to produce abutments that meet these machining parameters, the milling machine warns the operator of the need for component tool replacement. This approach ensures that the highest level of machining precision is consistently maintained for each milled abutment.

Milling Zirconia

Today, more abutments are being manufactured out zirconia than ever before. This is due to the fact that when zirconium is stabilized with yttrium trioxide (Y_2O_3) it has excellent mechanical properties for intra-oral use. It behaves very similarly to stainless steel, while its color can be modified to mimic the colors of teeth. Stabilized zirconia has a flexural strength of around 1200–1300 MPa, which compares well with PFM's flexural strength of around 1400 MPa. It also resists cyclical loading stresses very well (Piconi and Maccauro 1999). Zirconia has been shown to be kinder to the peri-implant tissues than titanium as it creates less of an inflammatory reaction (Warashina et al. 2003; Degidi et al. 2006). This combination of strength characteristics, tooth color compatibility, and soft tissue acceptance, makes zirconia a very desirable material for custom abutment fabrication.

Milling of zirconium is similar to that of titanium; long dime-sized rods of *non-sintered* zirconia are employed (Figure 6.12).

Zirconia is best milled in a non-sintered state (known as the *green state*) as fully sintered Zirconia is so hard, making milling difficult and detrimental to the mechanical properties of the finished abutment. Alternatively, when zirconia is milled *before* full sintering, the useful mechanical properties of the material are preserved. The sintering process induces a 20% *sintering shrinkage* which must be allowed for in the abutment design to obtain a properly fitting abutment (Manicone et al. 2007). Zirconia abutments are therefore designed 20% larger than the desired final abutment (Figures 6.13 and 6.14).

A green-state milled abutment is sintered beginning at 500°C up through a range of temperatures to 1200–1500°C. This temperature range increases crystalline formation for maximum density without creating an excess of porosity formation. Sintering temperatures above 1500°C cause the porosity of the grains to increase so that it becomes impossible to produce a high-density abutment (Karaulov and Kudyak 1975).

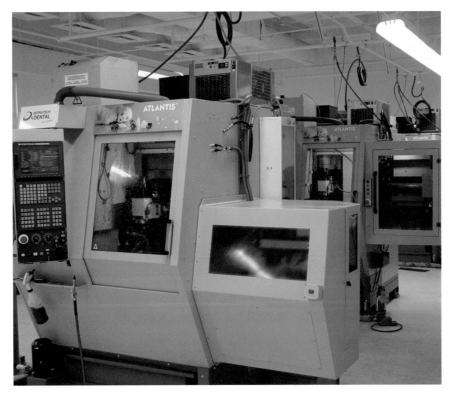

Figure 6.9 Typical milling machinery.

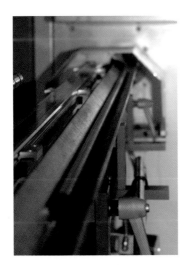

Figure 6.10 A long titanium rod, seen here entering the milling chamber, can be milled into many different abutments.

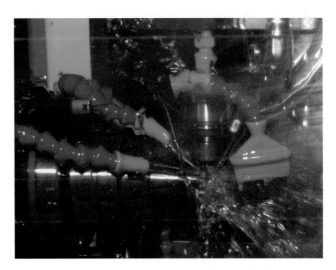

Figure 6.11 Water spray is employed to cool the cutting tools and titanium during the milling process.

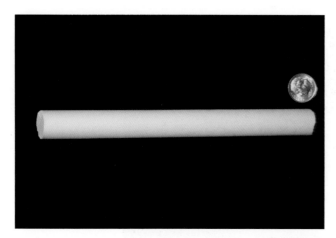

Figure 6.12   Dime-sized rods of zirconium are employed to create ceramic custom abutments.

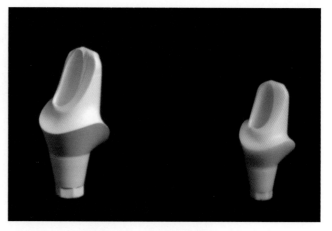

Figure 6.14   Different sizes of a central incisor abutment made of zirconia before (larger) and after (smaller) sintering.

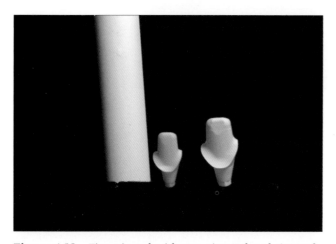

Figure 6.13   Zirconia rod with non-sintered and sintered central incisor abutments.

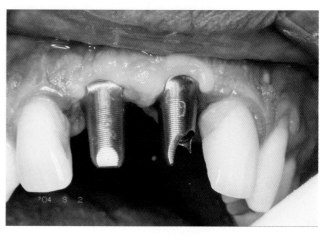

Figure 6.15   Machined and finished gold hue abutments with surface retentive grooves.

Once sintered, a zirconia abutment is finished and ready for intra-oral use.

Finishing Metallic Custom Abutments

Depending upon the system employed, finishing procedures of the various abutment manufacturing processes differ considerably. Metal finishing can range from hand polishing and contouring the raw titanium, to where abutments are milled into a finished state with retentive grooves and surface anatomy (requiring no surface smoothness corrections). Computer-guided surface finishing procedures can create superior surface characteristics to those obtainable with hand polishing methods. Figures 6.15 and 6.16 illustrate a comparison of a finished machined abutment surface to a manually polished abutment surface. Titanium can be coated with titanium nitride (TiN) to convert a sliver-colored abutment to a gold hue. TiN is a ceramic material that adheres to a titanium abutment by a vapor deposition process.

One advantage of using a gold hue surface application can be seen in the esthetic zone when there is thin tissue and the clinician employs a titanium abutment. A silver-colored titanium abutment can discolor the gingival margin, thus compromising the esthetic results of a visible implant restoration (Figure 6.17a). With the gold hue this problem is markedly improved as its yellow color does not discolor the gingival tissues (Figure 6.17b). Additionally, gold hue abutments can be used underneath all-ceramic crowns so that the underlying silver-colored metallic abutment does not lower the intrinsic value of the overlying crown (Figure 6.17c).

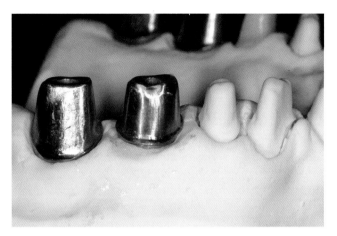

Figure 6.16 Hand polished titanium abutments.

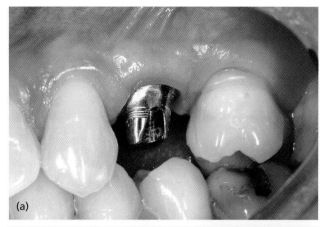

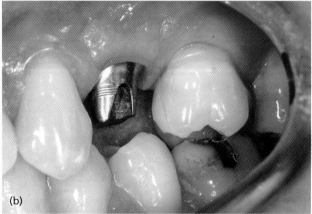

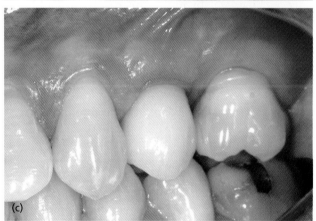

Another advantage of coating an abutment with TiN is that the coating withstands surface damage from routine intra-oral hygiene procedures better than uncoated abutments (Mengel et al. 2004). Mechanical abrasion by sharp dental hygiene instruments can leave more pronounced indentations and roughness on non-coated abutments when they are compared to silver nitride-coated abutments. These data suggest that TiN-coated abutment bases would be a better long-term plaque resister through the life of the implant prosthesis (due to better surface smoothness preservation), than would uncoated abutment bases.

Zirconium abutments are "finished" by the sintering process. Surface treatments and mechanical abrasion techniques to polish, smooth, or reshape the finished abutment can weaken the physical properties of the material and, therefore, are contraindicated.

Custom Abutment Inspection

Abutment Inspection is an ongoing, automated process that takes place at all stages during the virtual abutment design. Numerous proprietary *virtual tools* continuously monitor abutment features such as:

* Margin depth (facial, lingual, mesial, and distal).
* Margin width.
* Occlusal clearance.
* Proximity to neighboring teeth and interproximal contact point locations.
* Core thickness and height.
* Base shape.
* Screw access.
* Cuspal morphology.

During each stage of the design, these abutment features are optimized by software tools that relate the

Figure 6.17 (a) The gray color from a premolar titanium abutment can discolor the gingival tissues. (b) Improved tissue color with a gold hue replacement abutment. (c) Gold hue abutment under an all-ceramic crown.

abutment spatially to the future restored tooth by considering the following:

* Available edentulous space dimensions.
* Height of neighboring cusps, their cuspal angles, and the buccolingual and mesiodistal positions of those same cusps.

- Occlusal contours of the opposing teeth.
- Locations of neighboring contact points.
- Soft tissue margin height and contour of the periodontium of neighboring teeth.
- Morphology of the contralateral counterpart tooth.

Tools within the design software measure these variables so as to position the abutment within the ideal anatomic location while optimizing its contours to the anatomy of the surrounding structures.

The design software also contains abutment feature "*safety parameters*" that are based upon biomechanic and engineering principles. These design controls insure that during the virtual design process, the software will highlight areas where the design could be compromised. Such areas will not be "allowed" by the software control to be fabricated within the final abutment.

Manual Inspection

Once milled, rigorous manual inspection procedures are performed under magnification of the custom abutments. All aspects of the abutment are inspected so that the fit into the connection is accurate, there are no visible nicks and scratches on the surface, the margins are sharply defined, easily readable, and at the proper gingival height, and that the occlusal clearance is adequate. In multi-unit cases, all abutments are checked for proper parallelism and path of insertion. If any one of these inspected abutment aspects is deemed unsatisfactory, the abutment is rejected and remade.

Key aspects of metallic abutment manual inspection

- Machine surface finish
- Fit of the abutment interface
- Geometric inspection
- Presence of burrs and surface irregularities
- Comparison of the manufactured abutment to approved virtual abutment design
- Complete coverage of the abutment with the TiN coating

Inspection features specific to Zirconia abutments

- Proper color and shade
- Inspection for surface defects

It is interesting to note that, due to the high level of control that virtual design and virtual inspection procedures employ, combined with ongoing proprietary software enhancements, production flow process improvements, and manufacturing process improvements, the internal abutment "rejection rate" is reportedly kept at <2%.

Ordering an Atlantis Patient-specific Abutment

When ordering Atlantis VAD software-designed abutments, a critical series of abutment design parameters must be provided by the clinician to the dental laboratory so that the final abutment is correctly designed. The use of the clinician-to-laboratory prescription order form specifically designed for Atlantis orders can enhance (and simplify) this process. Although default values exist for abutment features (i.e. the buccal, distal, mesial, and lingual margin heights relative to the peri-implant sulcular margin height, and the differing abutment emergence width options) many abutment dimension values can be customized by the clinician to create an ideal final abutment.

The *clinician-to-laboratory prescription form* (Figure 6.18) presents the differing abutment design options for customization, and facilitates communication between the clinician and the dental laboratory. Once the form is completed with the clinician's design preferences, it is sent to the laboratory along with the standard laboratory form, implant-level impression, and case materials (Figure 6.19).

In addition to the preferences found on a standard laboratory work form, the key Atlantis abutment specifications requiring clinician input are as follow.

- *Implant brand/type:* The tooth number, implant brand, and specific platform measurement must be provided for each implant to be restored.
- *Duplicate abutment:* A functionally identical duplicate of the original Atlantis abutment can be ordered (not available in zirconia) and delivered together with the original abutment. Duplicate abutments can be used to serve as a master die to enhance laboratory accuracy and optimized crown fit, and eliminates the need for clinicians to remove the abutment placed in the patient's mouth to install the final restoration.
- *Restoration type:* Atlantis abutments are available for cement-retained and screw-retained (single tooth only) restorations.
- *Splinted restorations:* Splinting should be accurately indicated so that all abutments can be made perfectly parallel. A major advantage of software-designed splinted abutments is that the case parallelism, and axial wall taper, can be precisely matched unit to unit. Precision parallel design insures that retention of the splinted restoration is maximized, while providing the splint with a common path of insertion.

SECTION I: CUSTOMER INFORMATION

Please **PRINT** clearly. All information in Sections I and II are required. See case requirements on reverse side.

Today's Date   Patient Name or PO/Reference Number   Customer Number (if available)

Prescribing Clinician or Lab Signature: The signature below confirms that this product is being ordered at the request of a licensed dentist or on behalf of a licensed dentist whose information is on file with the lab.

Prescribing Clinician Zip Code (Required)

Shipping Preference
☐ Next Business Day PM (default)   ☐ 2-Day
☐ Next Business Day AM

Payment Method
☐ Invoice
☐ Am Ex   ☐ Visa   ☐ MasterCard
CC#: _____ Exp Date: _____

Ordered By (Name of Lab or Practice)

Bill To ☐ Same as "Ordered By"

Contact
Address
City   State   Zip
Phone   Fax
Email address:

Ship To ☐ Same as "Ordered By"   ☐ Same as "Bill To"

Contact
Address
City   State   Zip
Phone   Fax
Email address:

☐ **Send images and hold case.** (Case held until approval of abutment design images is provided.)   ☐ **Send images and process case.** (Images will be sent to "Ordered By" email address.)

SECTION II: CASE DATA

Please select from the Margin Position and Emergence Width Options to the right based on the type of case materials you are submitting:
- SILICONE Model of the Soft Tissue: Margin Position A, B or C; Emergence Width Option 1, 2, 3 or 4
- STONE Model of the Soft Tissue: Margin Position A, B or C; Emergence Width Option 4
- NO Model of the Soft Tissue: Margin Position B or C; Emergence Width Option 1, 2, 3 or 4

MARGIN POSITION

Select one option for how your margin position should be measured for the entire case:
☐ **A.** Margin position measured from gingival crest to abutment margin.
☐ **B.** Margin position measured from implant surface to abutment margin.
☐ **C.** Make abutment margin as close to interface as possible. No margin positions indicated.

B/F	D	M	L

EMERGENCE WIDTH OPTIONS

☐ **1. Full Anatomical Dimensions**
Largest diameter abutment provided with best emergence profile possible. A surgical incision for placement may be required.

☐ **2. Contour Soft Tissue** (default)
Medium diameter anatomically shaped abutment up to 1.0 mm larger than sulcus of model of soft tissue provided.

☐ **3. Support Tissue**
Anatomically shaped abutment will be up to 0.2 mm larger than sulcus of silicone model of soft tissue provided with desired emergence profile. "Easy" insertion.

☐ **4. No Tissue Displacement**
Abutment with no soft tissue support. **The abutment will not touch the soft tissue or stone model of the soft tissue provided.**

IMPLANT INFORMATION			ABUTMENT MATERIAL/TYPE				MARGIN DESIGN (select only one)		RETENTIVE SURFACE		HEALING ABUTMENT DIAMETER (in mm if present)
Tooth #	Implant brand & type	Platform diameter (in mm)	Abutment in titanium	Abutment in zirconia	GoldHue abutment	Gemini abutment	Chamfer	Shoulder	Yes	No	
			☐	☐	☐	☐	☐	☐	☐	☐	
			☐	☐	☐	☐	☐	☐	☐	☐	
			☐	☐	☐	☐	☐	☐	☐	☐	
			☐	☐	☐	☐	☐	☐	☐	☐	

PARALLEL ABUTMENTS (If final restorations will be splinted, **the abutments must be designed to be parallel to one another.**)
Will restorations be splinted? ☐ **No**   ☐ **YES** (Circle groups of abutments and/or teeth that will be splinted together.)

1 2 3 4 5 6 7 8 9 10 11 12 13 14 15 16
32 31 30 29 28 27 26 25 24 23 22 21 20 19 18 17

Figure 6.18 Clinician-to-laboratory prescription form.

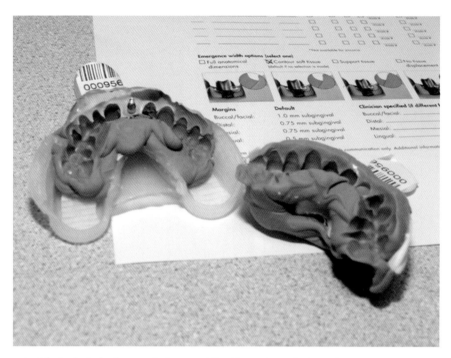

Figure 6.19   Case materials included when ordering an Atlantis custom abutment.

- *Abutment material:* The clinician can select their material of choice of either titanium, gold-shaded titanium (titanium with a thin coating of biocompatible TiN), or zirconia (available in up to five shades, including a translucent zirconia in white for screw-retained restorations).
- *Surface design:* A custom abutment can be milled with smooth axial walls or with retentive grooves milled into the axial walls (see Figure 6.15). The preference of the clinician dictates this choice, but if the abutment is short due to high placement and a lack of interocclusal clearance, retentive grooves will improve retention of the final restoration.
- *Margin design:* While default margin height values are provided and can be used, the clinician can define the subgingival depth of each margin. Routinely, the facial margin is placed 1–1.5 mm subgingival to hide the future crown margin under the tissue. The default values for the mesial, lingual, and distal margins can also be customized by the clinician. These margins can be placed higher in the tissue than the facial margin as they are not directly involved in case esthetics.

Implant placement depth into the bone can compromise margin placement, such that "high placements" result in margin depth limitations where the margin is required to be just above the implant–abutment connection. Proper implant placement depth generally leaves a 3 mm tall soft tissue collar above the platform, which aids in idealizing the facial margin's subgingival placement in the esthetic zone.

- *Emergence width options:* Here the clinician is given choices about how the abutment interacts with its surrounding soft tissue. The options range from no tissue displacement at all – resulting in no tissue blanching where the abutment easily passes by the tissue to seat into the implant – to a fully anatomic abutment design that often requires a soft tissue incision for it to be placed into the implant (Figure 6.20).

Emergence Width Options

No Tissue Displacement   Here the abutment base fits inside the peri-implant tissue without contacting the tissue (Figure 6.21).

Depending on the sulcus dimensions, there are wide and narrow designs available to the clinician. The no tissue displacement option is very useful in non-esthetic areas where tissue resistance can make abutment placement difficult (e.g. an upper second molar implant). By not applying any tissue pressure on insertion, this soft tissue design makes placing the abutment into the implant simple for the clinician.

The disadvantage of this design, despite its passive abutment seating, is that it often results in narrow abutments with small diameters. This occurs because the peri-implant sulcular cross-sectional dimensions are usually much smaller than the dimensions of the tooth requiring replacement. With a small-diameter sulcus the axial bulk of this type of abutment is often compromised, limiting many abutment shape-retentive features. Additionally, these small-diameter abutments

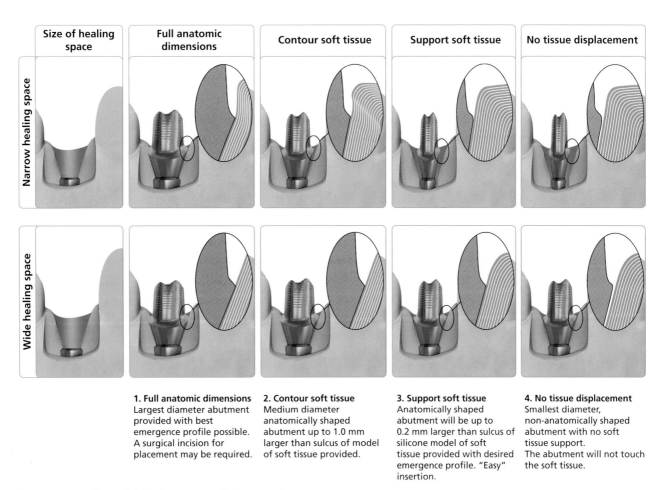

Figure 6.20 All available abutment soft tissue options.

mean that normal tooth contours have to be achieved in the final restoration by deliberately overcontouring the final crown contours.

One method of creating a bulkier abutment when selecting this option is to use a wide-diameter healing cap after implant exposure so as to form a wide-diameter sulcus as the tissue heals around the healing cap. This will form a wider sulcus, which will allow the use of a wider design for more abutment bulk, without applying pressure to the surrounding soft tissues.

Support Soft Tissue Here the abutment base rests against the peri-implant tissues, compressing them at the most by 0.2 mm, and filling the sulcus completely without blanching the tissues (Figure 6.22).

This design creates the desired soft tissue emergence profile without overcompressing the surrounding sulcular tissue. Utilizing an oversized healing cap will also improve abutment axial bulk when this soft tissue option is selected.

Contour Soft Tissue This abutment base compresses the surrounding soft tissue approximately 1 mm in all directions (Figure 6.23).

The clinician will face some soft tissue resistance when inserting this abutment design. Anesthesia is often required to be able to screw these abutments completely into the implant as patients can experience pain while seating the abutment. The advantage to this design is that it begins to create a more anatomic abutment morphology (without requiring a surgical placement) when compared with the previous two designs.

Full Anatomic Dimensions The fully anatomic abutment design attempts to reproduce the lost tooth's original size and morphology (Figure 6.24).

The advantage of this design is that the final crown can be created with an ideal anatomic form because the underlying abutment is full sized and recreates a near-perfect tooth preparation for the crown to mate with. The disadvantage is that it often needs to be placed surgically. However, recent design

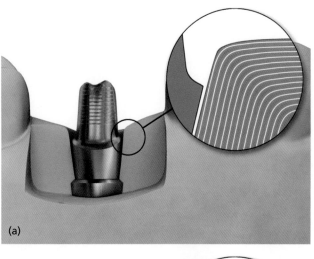

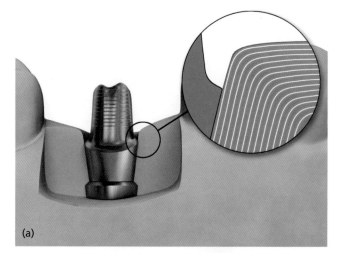

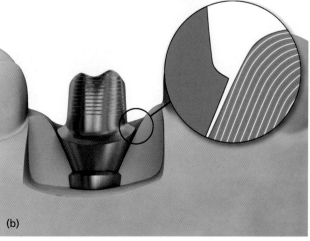

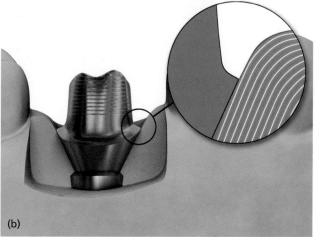

Figure 6.21 (a) No tissue displacement with a narrow abutment base design. (b) No tissue displacement with a wide abutment base design.

Figure 6.22 (a) Support soft tissue with a narrow abutment base design. (b) Support soft tissue with a wide abutment base design.

improvements have made it possible to place anatomic abutments non-surgically by incorporating new base features that induce peri-implant *sulcular stretching* when the abutment is screwed into place.

The specific geometric anatomic considerations can be optimized and customized for each individual patient's counterpart tooth. This is done by matching the total dimensions of the tooth to be replaced. The matching counterpart tooth (i.e. counterpart tooth no. 9 with implant in the no. 8 site) is measured in all dimensions and "mirror imaged" to create a virtual crown that fits into the implant site (Figure 6.25).

The virtual crown is then redrawn in a "mesh view" (see Figure 6.8f) so that beneath it a fully anatomic abutment is virtually created (Figure 6.26).

The counterpart tooth and the virtual crown guide the design of the fully anatomic abutment morphology.

ABUTMENT PLACEMENT USING SULCULAR STRETCHING

It is often difficult to create naturally appearing soft tissue contours that neighbor implant abutments. Implant platforms and healing caps are often much smaller than the tooth to be replaced. This may result in resorption of height and width of the alveolar ridge. After integration and soft tissue healing, a peri-implant sulcus forms around the shape of the healing cap (Figure 6.27). For an optimal gingival contour of the final crown, such a sulcus needs to be reduced or eliminated. Regardless of the implant or healing cap diameter, the peri-implant sulcus shape must usually be altered for the final restoration to appear natural.

Attempts to contour tissue have included the use of provisional restorations to form the desired soft tissue

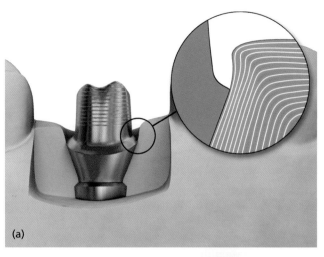

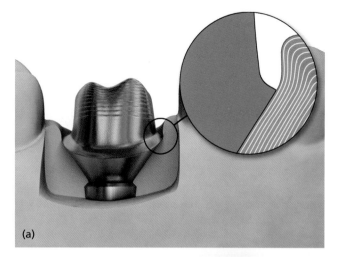

Figure 6.23 (a) Contour soft tissue with a narrow abutment base design. (b) Contour soft tissue with a wide abutment base design.

Figure 6.24 (a) Fully anatomic dimensions with a narrow abutment base design. (b) Fully anatomic dimensions with a wide abutment base design.

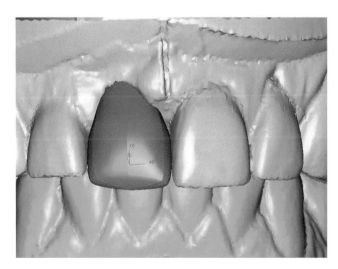

Figure 6.25 Virtual crown for tooth no. 8 to anatomically match tooth no. 9.

anatomy following stage II implant exposure surgery. One such procedure uses bonded (to neighboring teeth), properly shaped, provisional pontics that apply pressure to the peri-implant tissue over the implant (Kois and Kan 2001; Kim et al. 2009). Another uses abutments that support overcontoured provisional crowns to push out the tissue as it heals (Touati et al. 1999; Pow and McMillan 2004; Spyropoulou et al. 2009). Yet another uses the extracted natural tooth to sculpt the tissues that the tooth was just removed from (Margeas 2006).

As the tissue matures around these provisional alternatives, it takes on the shape of the gingival portion of the tooth, pontic, or provisional crown. Before implant prosthodontics became mainstream, this molding of the tissue was routinely utilized in the anterior region to approximate the appearance of a pontic emerging from the ridge in the way that a natural tooth emerges from the free gingival margin.

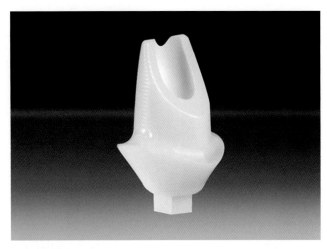

Figure 6.26   Fully anatomic finished zirconia abutment.

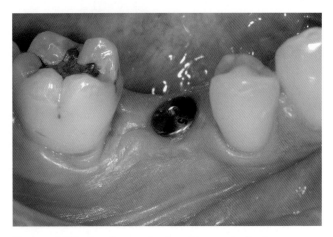

Figure 6.27   Small round sulcus that typically forms around the healing cap.

Today, this ridge tissue preparation method has been adapted to form ideally shaped peri-implant sulci.

When a provisional crown is used to sculpt the peri-implant sulcus, it must be overcontoured above the implant body. This will push out the lateral walls of the sulcus, widening it into an ideal gingival shape (Figure 6.28). The final crown must also be overcontoured to maintain the matured tissue shape.

Unfortunately this technique conflicts with advice given for natural tooth restoration due to the undesirable gingival tissue response to overcontouring (Koth 1982; Jacques et al. 1999; Knoernschild and Campbell 2000; Yotnuengnit et al. 2008). As an alternative to using overcontoured provisional crowns, it is possible to employ fully anatomic custom abutments to shape the tissues (Kerstein et al. 2000). These abutments can be waxed and cast in gold or digitally designed and CAD/CAM machine milled out of titanium or zirconia (Figure 6.29).

Sulcular stretching CAD/CAM abutments are designed to passively fill the healing cap-shaped sulcus from the top of the implant up to 2 mm below the subcrestal tissue. The outcropped abutment shoulder region helps create the dimensions and shape of the tooth to be replaced (Figure 6.30).

When this outcropped abutment design is screwed into place, the outcropping pushes the crestal third of the sulcus laterally to widen the sulcus around the abutment contours. The applied lateral pressure on the sulcus walls forces the sulcular tissue to conform to the abutment base shape. The sulcus is thereby forced to take on the abutment's outer morphology as its inner wall morphology (Figure 6.31).

This abutment seating procedure results in significant tissue blanching as the sulcular tissue is stretched. The blanching generally resolves within 1–2 days following abutment placement. Multiple clinical trials since 2008 have utilized such abutments and have shown that healthy tissue that has no inflammation quickly forms as the tissue adapts to the abutment's base shape. No significant recession around the abutments has been seen either. The final crown can then be made with full anatomic contours.

Where overcontouring implant restorations are used, the surrounding tissues respond poorly, frequently resulting in inflammation and alteration of the normal soft tissue architecture after a period of 42–49 days (Koth 1982; Yotnuengnit et al. 2008). Overcontoured crown margins demonstrate poor emergence profiles that blanch the gingival margin (due to pressure) and compromise periodontal health. Clinicians and lab technicians now aim to control the emergence profile of crowns on natural teeth in order to limit recession and crown margin exposure (Knoernschild and Campbell 2000).

Fully anatomically designed abutments, on the other hand, can effectively shape the tissues without recession and inflammation, despite initial tissue blanching, because the peri-implant tissue is actually *edentulous ridge tissue*. Edentulous ridge tissue does not react to applied pressure in the same way that gingival tissue reacts. The response of edentulous ridge peri-implant tissue to sulcular stretching mirrors that of its adaptation to a pressurized bridge pontic.

The simplicity of using anatomically shaped abutment designs to create ideal sulcular shapes around implant abutments, offers significant advantages to both the clinician and patient. The clinician simply has to screw in a properly designed, "outcropped" abutment shape, in the same fashion as any restorative implant component (e.g. impression coping, temporary or stock abutment, healing cap) is placed intra-orally. This eliminates the need for releasing incisions during abutment placement, which minimizes patient

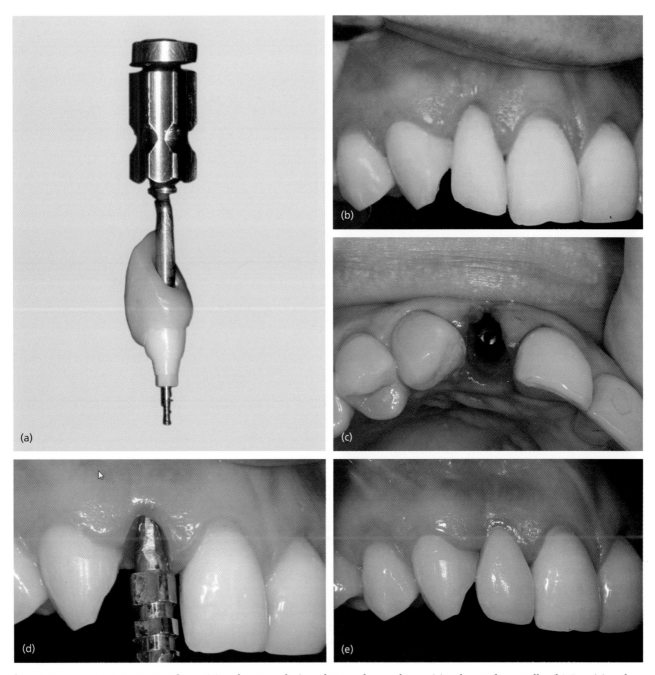

Figure 6.28   (a) Overcontoured provisional crown designed to push out the peri-implant sulcus walls. (b) Provisional crown in place. (c) Widened peri-implant sulcus. (d) Impression coping in place. (e) Final crown in place with nicely shaped esthetic gingival contours.

trauma, suture removal, postoperative discomfort, and healing time.

Many restorative practitioners are unwilling to perform releasing incision surgery. They may be more likely to use undersized abutments, small-based custom abutments, and stock abutments – all of which lack the anatomic form required to reproduce a life-like final gingival margin shape. The ease of placement of a sulcular stretching abutment makes them an attractive alternative to performing the releasing incisions routinely required to place an anatomic abutment. The use of sulcular stretching offers a simplified procedure from which to obtain ideal sulcular contours regardless of the healing cap dimensions. The principles of sulcular stretching will be discussed in more detail later in the next section on clinical cases.

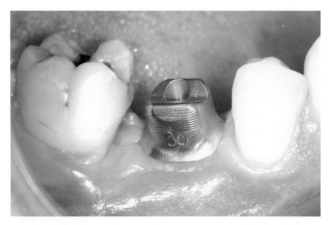

Figure 6.29 Gold hue abutment that was used to stretch the peri-implant sulcus of tooth no. 30 into natural first molar gingival contours.

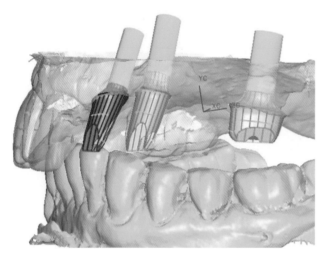

Figure 6.30 Software design images of outcropped shoulder regions of anatomic abutments in the nos 10, 11, and 14 sites.

CLINICAL EXAMPLES

CAD/CAM Designed Custom Abutments

The following clinical cases mainly use Atlantis abutments. This is because Atlantis abutments can work seamlessly with many of the available implant systems, which offers the restoring clinician a great deal of flexibility. Additionally, Atlantis virtual design technology can first create a healing abutment. Later in the course of the treatment, it can also alter the healing abutment contours to better fit the soft tissue changes that occur during surgical healing. This affords the clinician a predictable way to insure ideal clinical end results after the peri-implant tissues mature around a healing abutment. No other available abutment system can redesign duplicate abutments with subtle improved contour

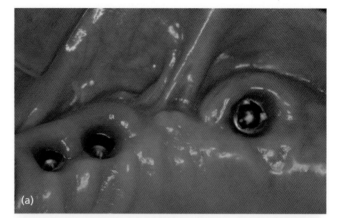

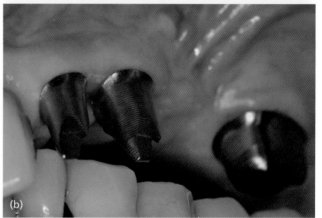

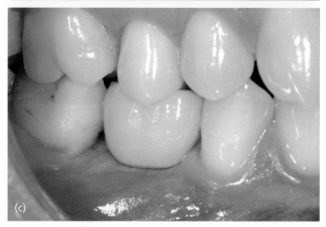

Figure 6.31 (a) Uncovered implants in the sites shown in Figure 6.30 with rounded peri-implant sulci. (b) Three gold hue abutments in these sites, stretching the sulci into an improved anatomic shape. (c) Final crowns in place.

variations without recreating an entirely new abutment for scanning. Virtual design recontouring makes changing a healing abutment made of titanium with a perfected second abutment milled out of another material (e.g. gold hue or zirconia), a highly efficient, predictable, and simple clinical process.

The other clinical cases presented here are of a Procera single unit zirconia abutment, and of a Straumann Etkon complex implant prosthesis.

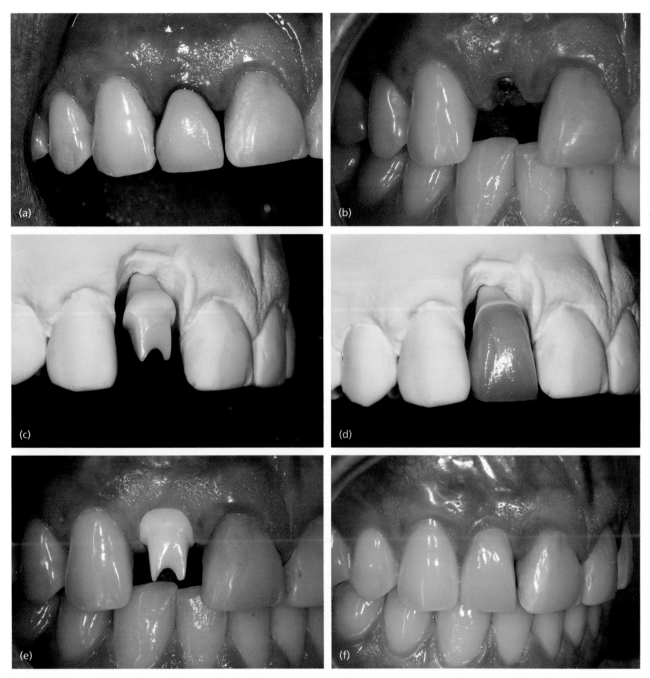

Figure 6.32 (a) Failing lateral incisor that had been restored with a PFM crown. (b) An Astratech implant placed into the residual edentulous ridge with the healing cap partially covered by soft tissue. (c) Zirconia abutment fitted to the master cast. (d) All-ceramic restoration created on the abutment. (e) Zirconia abutment screwed into place. (f) Final crown cemented over the abutment.

Clinical Case 1: Atlantis Zirconia Abutment Where the Final Crown and Custom Abutment Were Fabricated After Stage I Healing

An Atlantis custom abutment (and the final crown) can be fabricated to completion, in advance of their clinical insertion, from one scanned master cast. The abutment and crown fabrication can be inserted as soon as the implant has osseointegrated and is ready for restoration. This case also illustrates the simplicity of creating ideal gingival contours from a very small peri-implant sulcus using the sulcular stretching technique (Figure 6.32).

A failing, endodontically treated, lateral incisor (tooth no. 7) had been previously restored with a PFM crown. Following extraction and socket healing, an

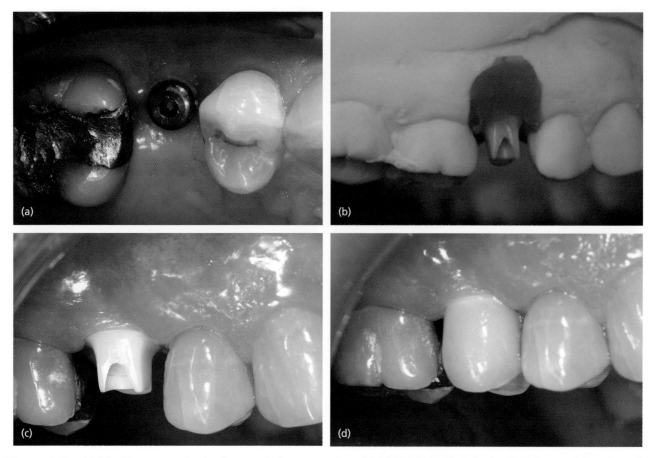

Figure 6.33 (a) Maxillary premolar implant ready for restoration. (b) Master cast after the implant impression was made with the wax-up sleeve. (c) Procera abutment seated intra-orally. (d) Final all-ceramic crown placed between teeth no. 3 and no. 5.

implant was placed into the residual edentulous ridge. The healing cap was partially covered by soft tissue.

When healing was complete, implant impression procedures were accomplished, and a master cast was fabricated and scanned into the design software. An Atlantis zirconia abutment (AAZ™, Astratech/Atlantis) was designed virtually and then milled and fit to the master cast. The final all-ceramic restoration was then created on this zirconia abutment.

In one clinical session the healing cap was removed, the zirconia abutment screwed into place, and the final crown cemented over the abutment. Note the blanching of the peri-implant tissues that resulted from placing the fully anatomic abutment. This stretched out the very small preoperative sulcus into an optimal tissue shape. The mesial diastema between teeth no. 7 and no. 8 was artistically rendered to mimic the diastema between teeth no. 9 and no. 10.

Clinical Case 2: Single Unit Procera Zirconia Custom Abutment Using the Wax–Scan–Mill Method

Procera abutment fabrication can be done using the wax–scan–mill technique to create the final abutment (Figure 6.33). In this clinical case, a maxillary premolar Nobel Biocare implant for tooth no. 4 was ready for restoration following healing.

Implant impression procedures were completed and a master cast was fabricated. A wax-up sleeve was then set into place on the implant analog. An abutment was waxed into the desired morphology and was scanned and milled in zirconia and screwed into place intra-orally. A zirconia coping was manufactured, to which the porcelain was applied. The finished crown was then installed between teeth no. 3 and no. 5.

A published comparison of Atlantis zirconia with Procera zirconia (Procera AllZirkon) illustrated some important differences between these two abutment materials (Kerstein and Radke 2008). The mean load to failure for the Atlantis abutment was higher than the Procera AllZirkon abutment although both materials were deemed strong enough for intra-oral use. A Weibull analysis determined that Atlantis abutment demonstrated a statistically significant higher probability of survival across the range of human occlusal loads. Lastly, the surface character of the Atlantis abutment appeared denser and less porous than the AllZirkon abutment in scanning electron micrograph material fracture images.

Clinical Case 3: Improving Tissue Color by Replacing an Atlantis Titanium Abutment with a Gold Hue Abutment

Because virtual design creates computer files of the abutment shape, differing abutments made from various materials can often be easily changed intra-orally as the prosthetic case requires. Titanium abutments used during surgical healing and early sulcus shape formation can be replaced with gold hue or zirconia abutments. The latter can be altered slightly to be better adapted to the gingival tissue margins, and to enhance the gingival margin color that approximates the final crown. This case reused virtual design files to allow the clinician to replace the abutment (Figure 6.34 and 6.35).

The patient had an Astratech implant in site no. 12 with a well-formed peri-implant sulcus shape that resulted from a correct implant depth and wide healing cap diameter. A virtual abutment was designed, milled in titanium, and seated intra-orally. Despite the tissue blanching that occurred around the titanium abutment after it was torqued into place and covered with a provisional crown, the silver-colored abutment discolored the gingival margin.

To compensate for this discoloration, a new gold hue replacement abutment was milled from the same digital design file and set into the master cast. The replacement gold hue abutment was inserted intra-orally, after which a final crown was fabricated on this abutment. Note the improved tissue color the gold hue abutment imparts to the gingival margin when compared with the titanium abutment.

Clinical Case 4: Complex Fixed Prosthesis Abutment Alteration for Zimmer Implants Prior to Final Restoration Fabrication

A complex fixed implant prosthesis containing many supportive abutments can also undergo abutment replacement by utilizing the multiple digital design files required to fabricate the first set of abutments.

This case shows how the first set of abutments used during provisionalization could be altered in the design process to create new zirconia abutments to improve abutment–tissue adaptation (Figure 6.36). These new abutments were then installed intra-orally and restored with a Lava prosthesis.

This patient had a full arch PFM restoration with poor esthetics. There was poor soft tissue adaptation in the gingival third around many of the prosthetic teeth. The patient presented with advanced periodontal disease requiring prosthesis and tooth removal.

After planning and implant placement, when healing was complete, a set of Atlantis titanium abutments were virtually designed, milled, and torqued into place in the nos 7, 9, and 10 sites. Note how the margins of these three abutments appear short of the true gingival margin. Although satisfactory for the provisionalization stage of this case, unless their margins were redesigned, these titanium abutments would negatively affect the esthetics of the final prosthesis.

This case was staged such that after the initial implants integrated, teeth nos 3, 6, 11, and 14 were then extracted and new implants placed into these extraction sites. After their integration, an impression was made to design abutments for the newly placed implants and to redesign the three original anterior abutments. All the required abutment changes were virtually designed on this new master cast. This meant that a set of replacement zirconia abutments could be milled, and then torqued into place intra-orally.

Note the improved margin–tissue adaptation of the three new zirconia abutments as compared with the previously problematic anterior titanium ones. The final prosthesis, made from a Lava bridge, when combined with the replacement zirconia abutments, provided a vastly superior esthetic result when compared with the initial patient presentation.

Clinical Case 5: Atlantis Titanium Healing Abutment Alterations to Better Match the Contours of a Neighboring Prepared Tooth

The simplicity of the process of altering a healing abutment to better suit the final prosthesis can be seen in this case (Figure 6.37). Here, a single implant was used to replace tooth no. 8. An initial healing abutment was designed virtually, milled in titanium, and then placed intra-orally.

Tooth no. 9 was then prepared for a full coverage restoration. After preparation it was determined that the original titanium abutment was too small circumferentially when compared with the prepared tooth. If left, this circumferential abutment/prepared tooth size discrepancy would compromise the esthetics because

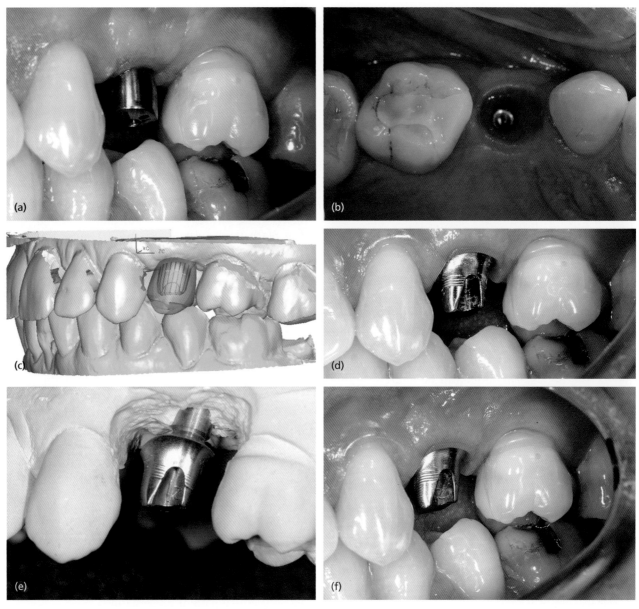

Figure 6.34 (a) Healing cap protruding through the soft tissue. (b) Astratech implant beneath the soft tissue. (c) Virtual design file of the abutment and crown. (d) An Atlantis titanium abutment in place within the implant. (e) A replacement gold hue abutment set into the master cast. (f) Replacement gold hue abutment placed intra-orally.

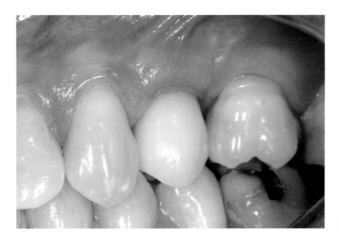

Figure 6.35 Final crown with improved tissue color.

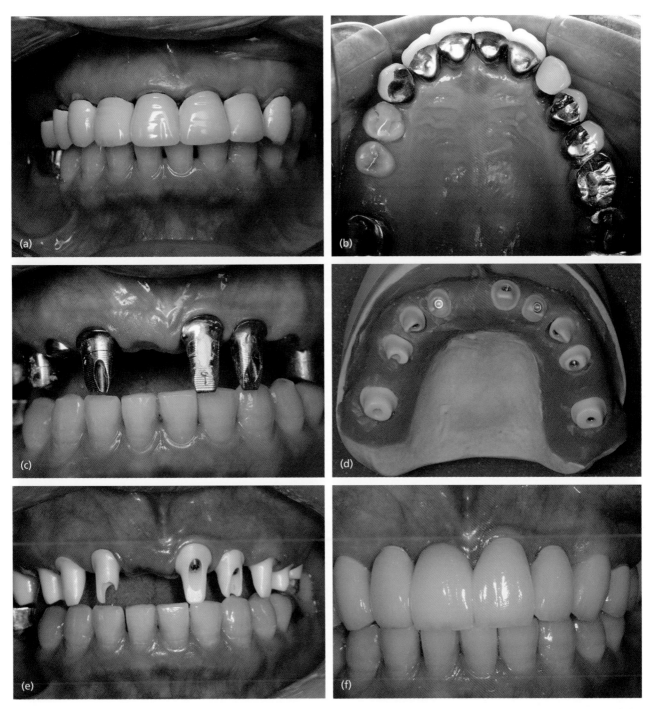

Figure 6.36 (a) A PFM full arch restoration with poor esthetics and poor soft tissue adaptation. (b) Occlusal view of the prosthesis. (c) Three titanium abutments in situ. (d) New master cast with all the required abutment changes. (e) Replacement zirconia abutments in place intra-orally with an improved margin–tissue adaptation. (f) Final Lava prosthesis.

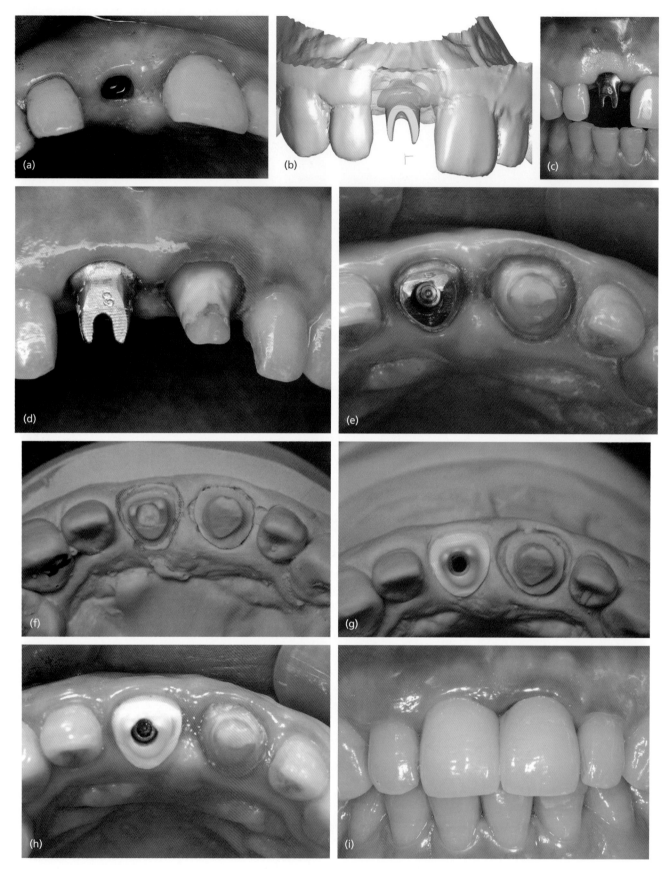

Figure 6.37 (a) Single Astratech implant. (b) Virtual design of the initial healing abutment. (c) Initial healing abutment placed intra-orally. (d) Tooth no. 9 prepared for full coverage. (e) Original titanium abutment, which was too small circumferentially compared with the prepared tooth. (f) Red outline showing the circumferential size change needed. (g) Redesigned zirconia abutment with a wider base dimension. (h) Equal-sized tooth preparations achieved with the new zirconia abutment. (i) Two crowns in place with comparable gingival base dimensions.

the two final crowns would be unmatched in the gingival contours.

The titanium abutment was outlined in red pencil on a stone model. This indicated the circumferential size changes needed to better match the abutment to the size of the prepared tooth. The outlined changes were then used to redesign a zirconia abutment that was properly matched in circumferential base dimension to the prepared no. 9 tooth.

Once the equally sized tooth preparations were in place, the final crowns were then fabricated and installed. Note the crown–gingival dimension equality that was made possible by improving the circumferential size matching. This was achieved by replacing the small titanium healing abutment with a properly sized zirconia abutment.

Clinical Case 6: Straumann Etkon Zirconia Abutments to Restore a Failing PFM Reconstruction

Straumann offers an alternative to the Atlantis approach with the Etkon Abutment System (Figure 6.38). In this case, the patient was not esthetically pleased with the implant reconstruction that had been done.

The original crowns (placed upon Straumann implants) were removed. The implants were reimpressed with the appropriate Straumann impression copings that matched the differing implant sizes. A master cast was retrieved upon which the Etkon waxing sleeves were placed into the implant analogs inside the silicone key of the provisional restoration. Then, using silicone keys made from the provisional restoration, the abutment wax-ups were created.

Cast metal abutments were created for the posterior teeth, while zirconia abutments were created for the anterior teeth (Straumann does not offer posterior abutments in zirconia). Note that the overall posterior abutment morphology resulting from the wax-up technique did not anatomically compare to the abutment morphology created by Atlantis virtual design software.

The anterior wax-ups were scanned, milled, and placed back onto the master cast. There was poor gingival adaptation of the milled abutments, such that some of the facial and interproximal margins were supragingival. The original anterior wax-up that was scanned and milled had a proper abutment–gingival margin adaptation, indicating that the Etkon scanning and/or milling processes created a distortion of the original abutment contours. To compensate for this distortion, pink porcelain was applied to the base area of the abutments to hide the whitish zirconia color.

The zirconia abutments were installed intra-orally, and the no. 7 abutment fractured slightly during screw tightening (Figure 6.38k). The zirconia copings were then designed and milled. These copings were veneered with porcelain to create the final crowns. Note how the pink porcelain helped to blend the final result into the surrounding tissues.

The need for pink porcelain in this Etkon case demonstrates how the correction versatility of the Atlantis virtual design technology is a superior approach to that of the wax–scan–mill method of abutment manufacture. By altering the digital files to compensate for poor abutment–soft tissue adaptation (see Clinical cases 4 and 5), a non-ideal abutment can be easily improved to better meet the clinical requirements of the patient. This capability is only possible because of virtual design, which the wax–scan–mill methodology cannot offer the clinician.

Sulcular Stretching

Principles

When peri-implant sulcular tissue has an undersized healing cap, sulcular stretching can be clinically employed to change its shape. The aim is to alter the size and form of the sulcular tissue to the base shape of an outcropped fully anatomic abutment (see Figure 6.32). Clinical cases 7 and 8 illustrate the technique of sulcular stretching.

The *non-surgical placement* technique of a CAD/CAM abutment has a number of advantages. It results in the formation of ideal gingival contours and natural appearing implant restorations shortly after the fully anatomic abutment is screwed into place. It is preferable to stage II surgical anatomic abutment insertion using releasing incisions for both the patient and the clinician. For the patient there are less surgical procedures, decreased postoperative discomfort, reduced healing time, and no suture removal. The clinician simply screws into place a properly designed abutment shape once implant osseointegration is complete.

Indications for sulcular stretching

- The platform of the implant must be at least 2.5 mm below the soft tissue crest.
- The peri-implant sulcus should be significantly smaller than the tooth to be replaced.
- The implant fixture should be in the middle or lingual third of the ridge crest.
- The edentulous ridge should be well formed with the crestal height comparable to that of the neighboring teeth.
- Any preprosthetic tissue grafting, bone grafting, or ridge distraction (if required) should have all healed to completion with an implant fixture in place.

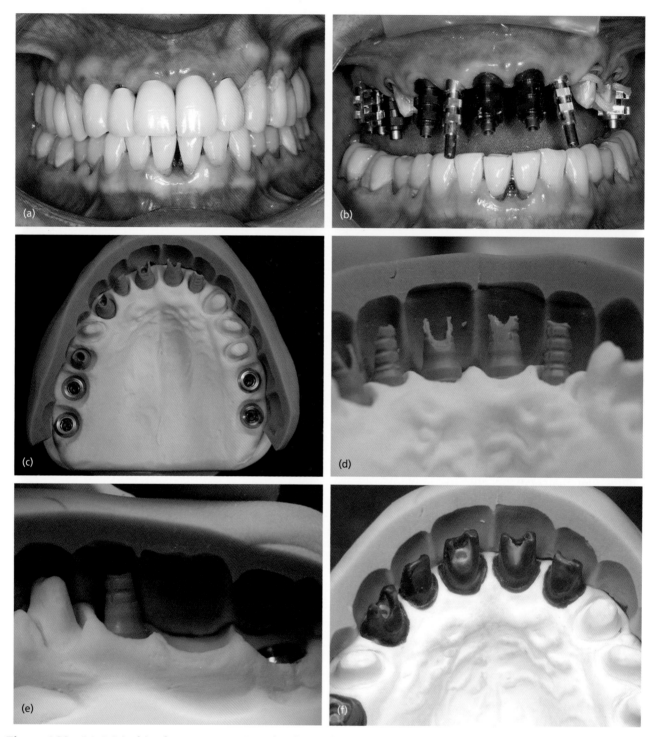

Figure 6.38 (a) Original implant reconstruction. (b) The implants were reimpressed with appropriate Straumann impression copings. (c) Master cast with Etkon waxing sleeves placed into the analogs. (d, e) Close-up of the anterior (d) and posterior (e) silicone keys. (f) Abutment wax-ups.

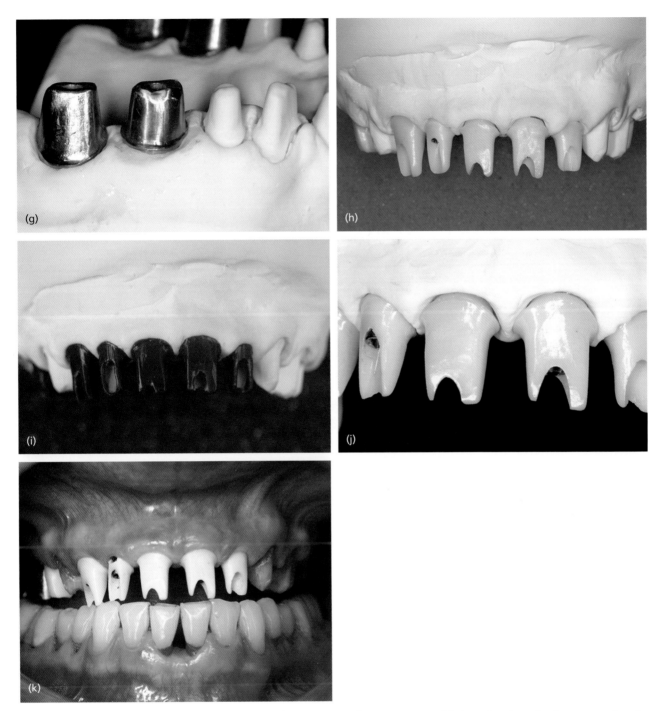

Figure 6.38 (*Continued*) (g) Cast metal posterior abutments on the master cast. (h) Anterior zirconia abutments placed back into the master cast showing poor gingival adaptation. (i) Anterior wax-up showing proper abutment–gingival margin adaptation. (j) Pink porcelain was applied to the base of the abutments to improve the final esthetic result. (k) Zirconia abutments placed intra-orally.

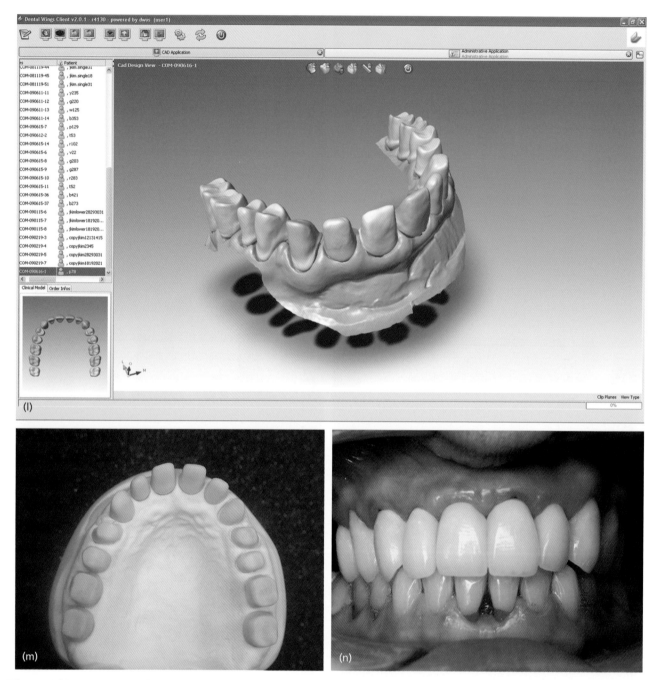

Figure 6.38 (*Continued*) (l) Zirconia copings being designed. (m) Zirconia copings were milled and placed onto the master cast for porcelain veneering. (n) Final crowns in situ.

Contraindications for sulcular stretching

- A high implant placement that results in <2.5 mm sulcus height.
- A labial one-third implant placement resulting in a very thin labial sulcular wall, which would likely be compromised from applied pressure resultant from stretching the tissue.
- Required preprosthetic surgical bone and soft tissue augmentation procedures have not been completed.

Site Preparation

Prior to the insertion of the outcropped fully anatomic abutment, the healing cap should be removed and the peri-implant sulcus anesthetized circumferentially. In this way the patient will be unaware of the applied pressure resulting from tightening the oversized abutment into place. If epinephrine is used, the peri-implant tissues will likely blanch white from vasoconstriction.

The abutment is then seated into the top of the implant by aligning and engaging the seating elements on the external or internal surfaces of the implant with the corresponding abutment seating features. This requires the operator to apply positive pressure against any tissue resistance encountered during the initial seating. Because the crestal sulcular tissue is under the abutment's outcropping, it will resist the initial seating somewhat, making it difficult to align the abutment with the implant seating elements.

Once the abutment is properly aligned and held down firmly, the screw should then be engaged into the implant. It should be torqued to place using the implant manufacturer's recommend torque wrench (up to 35 N-cm). While the abutment seats further and further into the implant, it will increasingly compress the tissues, thus turning them white. The fit should be verified radiographically and the provisional/final crown fabrication can then be undertaken.

An advantage of utilizing CAD/CAM patient-specific anatomic abutments is that the final crown can often be placed the same day as the abutment seating. This is because the crown can be made in advance, utilizing the abutment as the die for the final crown.

Clinical Case 7: Sulcular Stretching with an Anatomically Designed Abutment Base and Preparation Shoulder Morphology

Sulcular stretching can be achieved using an anatomically designed abutment base and preparation shoulder (Figure 6.39). In this case, an undersized healing cap had been placed into the implant in the no. 8 site. It did not in any way match the root morphology, gingival shape, or approximate width and breadth of tooth no. 9. Additionally, the facial tissue ridge crest above the no. 8 implant was too broad and low when compared with the gingival margin shape of tooth no. 9. Together, all of these tissue morphology discrepancies would result in an obvious esthetic mismatch of the restored no. 8 implant to its counterpart central incisor tooth.

An anatomically designed zirconia abutment (AAZ, Astratech/Atlantis) was used that incorporated a broadening triangular base shape that was smallest at the implant connection and widest at the subshoulder area. This feature stretched the healing sulcus into the desired width. The abutment shoulder contoured and forced the sulcus crest into an arch-shaped gingival margin that was a mirror-image of tooth no. 9. The triangular shoulder of the milled abutment approximated the outline form of tooth no. 9. This meant that when the abutment was removed after the sulcus healed, the previously undersized sulcus would have

the same increasingly wider dimensions of the abutment base.

Note that the inner walls of the peri-implant sulcus (those in contact with the abutment base) demonstrated some irritation and redness, very similar to that observed under a pontic that continuously presses on edentulous ridge tissue. The outer crestal tissues, those not in contact with the abutment base, on the other hand, appeared non-inflamed and healthy.

With the final crown in place on the anatomically designed abutment, the crown and gingival contours of the implant restoration appeared morphologically similar to those of tooth no. 9.

The stretched sulcular peri-implant tissue provided a healthy and naturally appearing esthetic result that was created *non-surgically*, solely by screwing into place a properly designed abutment base shape.

Clinical Case 8: Sulcular Stretching with a One-Piece Zirconia Abutment and Crown

Sulcular stretching can also be achieved using a one-piece zirconia abutment–crown (Figure 6.40). In this case, when the healing cap in the no. 13 site was removed, a peri-implant sulcus was revealed where the gingival contours were smaller and rounder than those for teeth no. 12 and no. 14.

In addition, the facial gingival margin was very different to the facial cervical tooth structure of the neighboring teeth. This resulted in an obvious tissue height and shape discrepancy that would have resulted in a poor esthetic result.

The sulcus was stretched with an anatomic one-piece zirconia abutment–crown (Atlantis Crown Abutment) designed with an outcropped shoulder. In this way the tissue could be moved outward by the shape of the subshoulder portion of the abutment that outcrops significantly just below the crest of the sulcus. Notice how the outcropping of the subshoulder area approximated the size of the tooth to be replaced, such that the sulcular tissue was stretched to the same dimensions.

Using a one-piece abutment–crown succeeded in stretching the facial tissue to approximate the neighboring tissue contours much better. In this way it provided an esthetically pleasing, natural looking result.

ADVANTAGES OF CAD/CAM ABUTMENTS VERSUS REGULAR CAST CUSTOM ABUTMENTS

- Abutments are precision created by smart software requiring no lab technician skill or knowledge to obtain an optimally shaped custom abutment.

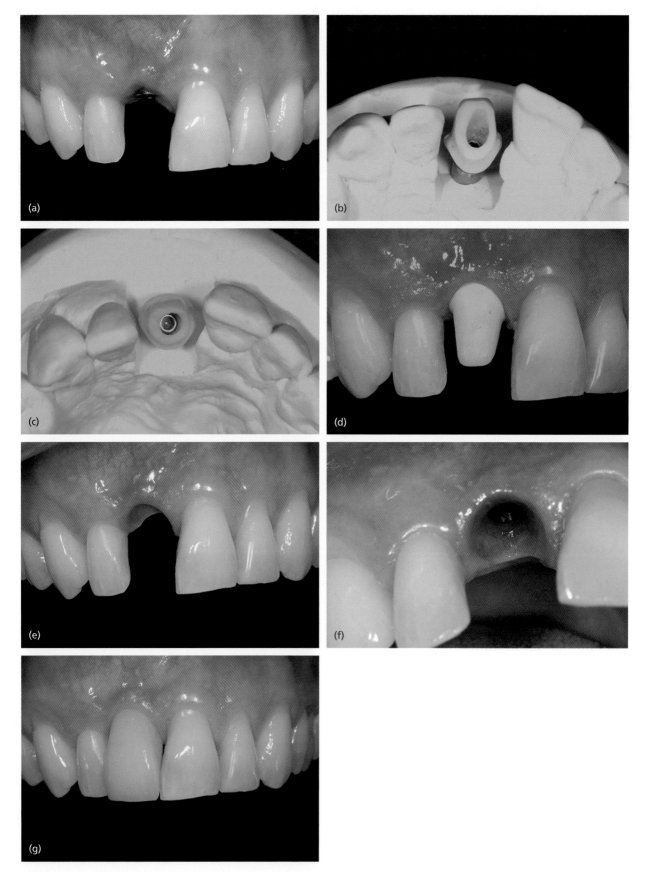

Figure 6.39 (a) Undersized healing cap of a no. 8 implant that is much smaller than the root area morphology of tooth no. 9. (b) Base shape and subshoulder designed to stretch the small sulcus (c) Incisal view of the abutment shoulder. (d) Ziconia abutment in situ. (e) Sulcular contours healed into an arch-shape. (f) Stretched and healed sulcus. (g) Final crown in place.

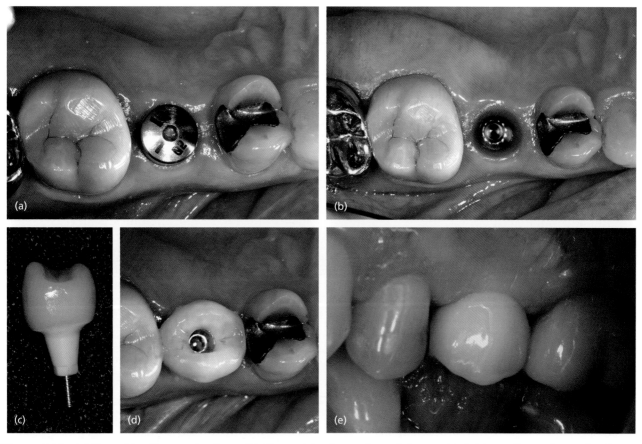

Figure 6.40 (a) Round healing cap in place. (b) The peri-implant sulcus of the no. 13 site is smaller and rounder than those of the neighboring teeth. (c) One-piece Atlantis zirconia crown–abutment with an outcropped subshoulder area. (d) Morphology of the no. 13 restoration closely resembling that of the neighboring teeth. (e) Final crown in place.

- The surface characteristics of a virtually design abutment are superior to cast abutments because each abutment is precision milled and highly mechanically polished.
- Each abutment is a one-piece entity with no abutment cylinder–alloy interface utilized. Therefore, abutments have higher mechanical tolerances for compromised implant placement alignment or when employed in tissue-deficient areas.
- It is easy to have precise duplicates made, giving the lab technician the exact shape of abutment that the patient needs. Duplicate abutments eliminate any inexact stone reproductions obtained through conventional impression procedures. Crown–abutment fit is therefore improved.
- Any compromised abutment contours can be virtually modified to improve the abutment regardless of abutment material used (e.g. zirconia, gold hue, titanium).
- Because the machining process is completely software driven and occurs irrespective of the chosen abutment material, any future abutment materials developed (e.g. lithium disilicate, composites) will easily fit into the manufacturing process.

COMMON PROBLEMS IN CAD/CAM ABUTMENT MANUFACTURING

The problems observed within abutment manufacturing depend on the chosen abutment solution.

1. For UCLA-type custom abutments:
   - Very labor intensive and requiring highly skilled technicians.
   - Difficult to ensure passive insertion and parallelism due to the need for wax-up.
   - Potential inconsistency of the final result due to the dependency on the individualized skill of the technician and the quality of the manual wax-up.

- There is a separation potential between a UCLA-type abutment and the cast metal if the latter is miscast.
- The cast interface is less precise than a milled interface for abutment fit into the implant.
- There is a potential for incurring an unpredictable cost per abutment due to the fluctuating prices of alloy materials.

2. For CAD/CAM solutions not including Atlantis virtual design:
   - Very labor intensive and requiring highly skilled technicians.
   - Difficult to ensure passive insertion and parallelism due to the need for wax-up.
   - Potential inconsistency of the final result due to the dependency on the individualized skill of the technician and the quality of the manual wax-up.
   - Most abutment systems create the final abutment utilizing an "inside-out approach" where the design focuses on the abutment rather than basing the design on the final tooth shape.
   - Traditional CAD utilizes individual "points" for adjusting abutment design that do not simultaneously result in improvement changes in other areas of the abutment.

In contrast to traditional CAD, the Atlantis virtual design software employs a *parametric design model* where appropriate changes in any one abutment contour will automatically alter related parameters, resulting in a cohesive abutment design.

CONCLUSIONS

State-of-the-art custom abutment manufacturing is a totally automated, computer-controlled process. It can produce esthetic, anatomic, and precise fitting custom abutments made out of differing dental materials. CAD/CAM has evolved in implant prosthodontics to be the leading method of custom abutment manufacturing available today. Although numerous implant companies offer CAD/CAM custom abutment solutions, the leading manufacturing process is the Atlantis VAD™ technology. This utilizes smart software, virtual tools, and internal system controls over the abutment design, milling procedures, and milling machinery. As a consequence it produces morphologically correct abutments that optimize clinically implanted tooth replacements.

This chapter details the entire process of custom abutment manufacture, from intra-oral impression procedures and master cast fabrication, through virtual abutment design, machine milling, surface finishing, and inspection of the final abutment.

Detailed information regarding the ordering of a custom abutment is also included because, within the ordering process, the clinician can input his/her own preferences. This means the custom abutment can meet their own specific clinical requirements.

Because custom abutments provide restoration support in the treatment of a wide range of differing clinical scenarios, select clinical cases have been included. Of special note is the recent development of a uniquely designed abutment that contains an outcropped base and subshoulder contour feature. The use of this can convert an undersized, peri-implant healing-cap-shaped sulcus into an ideal, anatomically shaped gingival margin. This can be achieved by simply screwing the abutment into place. All of these clinical cases illustrate the versatility and reliability of the Atlantis virtual abutment design process when compared with the wax–scan–mill abutment manufacturing process.

Acknowledgments

Special thanks to Ms Janie Shen of Astratech/Atlantis for her assistance in providing much of the included technical information.

REFERENCES AND ADDITIONAL READING

Andersson, M., Razzoog, M.E., Odén, A., Hegenbarth, E.A., & Lang, B.R. (1998). Procera: a new way to achieve an all-ceramic crown. *Quintessence International,* 29(5), 285–296.

Calamia, J.R. (1994). Advances in computer-aided design and computer-aided manufacture technology. *Current Opinion in Cosmetic Dentistry,* 1994, 67–73.

Degidi, M., Artese, L., Scarano, A., Perrotti, V., Gehrke, P., & Piattelli, A. (2006). Inflammatory infiltrate, microvessel density, nitric oxidesynthase expression, vascular endothelial growth factor expression, and proliferative activity in peri-implant soft tissues around titanium and zirconium oxide healing caps. *Journal of Periodontology,* 77, 73–80.

Drago, C.J. & Peterson, T. (2007). Treatment of an edentulous patient with CAD/CAM technology: a clinical report. *Journal of Prosthodontics,* 16(3), 200–208.

Eidenbenz, S., Lehner, C.R., & Scharer, P. (1994). Copy milling ceramic inlays from resin analogs: a practicable approach with CELAY system. *International Journal Prosthodontics,* 7, 134–42.

Isenberg, B.P. & Garber, D.A. (1994). Directly milled ceramic inlays and onlays CAD/CAM systems. In *Porcelain and Composite Inlays and Onlays: Esthetic Posterior Restorations,* ed. Garber, D.A. & Goldstein, R.E. Chicago: Quintessence, 143–155.

Jacques, L.B., Coelho, A.B., Hollweg, H., & Conti, P.C. (1999). Tissue sculpturing: an alternative method for improving esthetics of anterior fixed prosthodontics. *Journal of Prosthetic Dentistry*, 81(5), 630–633.

Karaulov, A.G. & Rudyak, I.N. (1975). Sintering zirconia with yttrium oxide. *Refractories and Industrial Ceramics*, 16(1/2), 123–127.

Kerstein, R.B., Castellucci, F., & Osorio, J. (2000). Utilizing computer generated titanium permanent healing abutments to promote ideal gingival form and anatomic restorations on implants. *Compendium*, 21(10), 793–802.

Kerstein, R.B. & Osorio, J. (2003). Utilizing computer generated duplicate titanium custom abutments to facilitate intraoral and laboratory implant prostheses fabrication. *Practical Procedures and Aesthetic Dentistry*, 15, 311.

Kerstein, R.B. & Radke, J. (2008). A comparison of fabrication precision and mechanical reliability of 2 zirconia implant abutments. *International Journal of Oral and Maxillofacial Implants*, 23(6), 1029–1036.

Kim, T.H., Cascione, D., & Knezevic, A. (2009). Simulated tissue using a unique pontic design: a clinical report. *Journal of Prosthetic Dentistry*, 102(4), 205–210.

Knoernschild, K.L. & Campbell, S.D. (2000). Periodontal tissue responses after insertion of artificial crowns and fixed partial dentures. *Journal of Prosthetic Dentistry*, 84(5), 492–498.

Kois, J.C. & Kan, J.Y. (2001). Predictable peri-implant gingival aesthetics: surgical and prosthodontic rationales. *Practical Procedures and Aesthetic Dentistry*, 13(9), 691–698.

Koth, D.L. (1982). Full crown restorations and gingival inflammation in a controlled population. *Journal of Prosthetic Dentistry*, 48(6), 681–685.

Manicone, P.F., Iommetti, P.R., & Raffaelli, L. (2007). An overview of zirconia ceramics: Basic properties and clinical applications. *Journal of Dentistry*, 35, 819–826.

Margeas, R.C. (2006). Predictable periimplant gingival esthetics: use of the natural tooth as a provisional following implant placement. *Journal of Esthetic and Restorative Dentistry*, 18(1), 5–12.

McLaren, E.A. & Sorensen, J.A. (1994). Fabrication of conservative ceramic restorations using copy milling technology. *Quintessence Journal of Dental Technology*, 17, 19–25.

Mengel, R., Meer, C., & Flores-de-Jacoby, L. (2004). The treatment of uncoated and titanium nitride-coated abutments with different instruments. *International Journal of Oral and Maxillofacial Implants*, 19(2), 232–238.

Nishimura, R.D., Chang, T.L., Perri, G.R., et al. (1999). Restoration of partially edentulous patients using customized implant abutments. *Practical Periodontics and Aesthetic Dentistry*, 11, 669–676.

Osorio, J. (1997). Customized dental abutment. United States Patent No. 5,674,069, October 7.

Osorio, J. & Ziegler, A. (1999). Customized dental abutments and methods of preparing or selecting the same. United States Patent No. 5,989,029, November 23.

Osorio, J. & Ziegler, A. (2001). Customized dental abutments and methods of preparing or selecting the same. United States Patent No. 6,231,342, May 15.

Piconi, C. & Maccauro, G. (1999). Zirconia as a ceramic biomaterial. *Biomaterials*, 20, 1–25.

Pow, E.H. & McMillan, A.S.A (2004). Modified implant healing abutment to optimize soft tissue contours: a case report. *Implant Dentistry*, 13(4), 297–300.

Spyropoulou, P.E., Razzoog, M., & Sierraalta, M. (2009). Restoring implants in the esthetic zone after sculpting and capturing the periimplant tissues in rest position: a clinical report. *Journal of Prosthetic Dentistry*, 102(6), 345–347.

Touati, B., Guez, G., & Saadoun, A. (1999). Aesthetic soft tissue integration and optimized emergence profile: provisionalization and customized impression coping. *Practical Periodontics and Aesthetic Dentistry*, 11(3), 305–314.

Warashina, H., Sakano, S., Kitamura, S., et al. (2003). Biological reaction to alumina, zirconia, titanium and polyethylene particles implanted onto murine calvaria. *Biomaterials*, 24, 3655–3661.

Yotnuengnit, B., Yotnuengnit, P., Laohapand, P., & Athipanyakom, S. (2008). Emergence angles in natural anterior teeth: influence on periodontal status. *Quintessence International*, 39(3), e126–133.

7
Relationship between Abutment Geometry and Peri-implant Tissue in Esthetic Zone Cases

Dean Morton, Tamer Abdel-Azim, and Wei-Shao Lin

Department of Oral Health and Rehabilitation, School of Dentistry, University of Louisville, Louisville, KY

INTRODUCTION

Dental implants have proven to be predictable long-term treatment options for optimizing the support, stability, and retention of dental prostheses. This has resulted in a greater acceptance of dental implants as important components of care by both patients and clinicians. There has been a concurrent rise in the expectations of optimal outcomes, both functional and esthetic.

In order to increase the predictability of a satisfactory treatment outcome, particularly from the esthetic perspective, provisional and definitive implant-based restorations must achieve several goals:

1. They must harmonize with the patient's overall appearance and face.
2. They must encourage a healthy intraoral environment.
3. They must imitate the natural appearance of the adjacent dentition by reproducing the form, size, texture, and optical properties of the teeth being replaced (Buser et al. 2004).

Successful contemporary dental implant treatment is therefore not only defined by the survival of implants or the absence of biologic and prosthetic complications, but also, and importantly, by an optimal esthetic outcome. The esthetic result must satisfy even the most demanding clinical circumstances and patient. Optimal three-dimensional positioning of the dental implants is determined by rigorous pretreatment diagnosis and planning. Restoration-driven treatment has, for the most part, been embraced to effectively reduce the risk of a negative esthetic or functional treatment outcome (Martin et al. 2007).

Factors contributing to the overall esthetic result may include the anatomy of the implant sites (gingival biotype, shape of adjacent teeth, bone level at adjacent teeth), placement of the implants (oral–facial position, mesial–distal position, coronal–apical position, distance between tooth–implant or implant–implant), the hard/soft tissue management procedures during the implant treatments, and the design or prosthetic management of provisional/definitive restorations. This chapter will focus on the prosthetic management of tissues adjacent to the dental implant via provisional restorations, customized impression techniques, and definitive abutments and final restorations.

PROVISIONAL RESTORATIONS PRIOR TO IMPLANT LOADING

General Considerations

Provisional restorations associated with implant therapy fall into two broad categories. First, there are those provisional restorations utilized between tooth extraction and implant placement/loading. Second, provisional restorations need to be supported by the implants subsequent to placement. Each form of provisional restoration plays a specific role in the achievement of satisfactory treatment results (Higginbottom et al. 2004).

The provisional restoration serves many purposes and provides several advantages when incorporated into dental implant-based treatments. Provisional restorations positioned subsequent to extraction and prior to implant placement provide patients with economic, esthetic, and functional replacements that are satisfactory in the short term. Provisional restorations used in this treatment phase should be durable and readily maintained. Further, they should lend themselves to simple removal and replacement, modification, and adjustment throughout the treatment process.

The clinician may also gather information relevant to the definitive treatment during the provisional restorative phase. This information may include tooth shade, restorative contours, and peri-implant soft tissue profile. Each of these parameters may also be used as a tool for communication between treatment team members, and between the treatment team and the patient. The ability of the patient to visualize and evaluate the proposed restorative outcome may be of great significance.

Soft and/or hard tissue augmentation is often an important aspect of the esthetics of implant-based treatment. Augmentation procedures may be undertaken to increase tissue volume, facilitating the placement of an implant and improving the likelihood of a stable long-term result. Augmentation procedures may be used to enhance esthetic conditions in areas where adequate volume for implant placement is present, but where the residual ridge contour is less than ideal from the esthetic perspective. Appropriately designed provisional restorations can enhance patient comfort and satisfaction during the lengthy healing periods associated with augmentation procedures. Further, duplicates of provisional restorations can allow the surgeon to visualize tissue deficits and the planned restorations.

Contouring of the proposed implant site can commence immediately following tooth extraction. The provisional restoration can be ovate in form to initiate the shaping of the future peri-implant soft tissue. This can be accomplished with removable or fixed provisional restorations, although removable provisional restorations should be used with caution, particularly in the presence of grafts.

Fixed provisional restorations offer several advantages in treatment based on dental implants. Fixed prostheses eliminate vertical pressure on the tissue, which is critical in protecting outcomes associated with augmentation procedures. Fixed provisional restorations are also associated with improved patient comfort and assessment of esthetic potential. Further, they may increase patient acceptance of implant treatment because of the satisfaction of psychologic demand. However, fixed provisional restorations often require longer chair time and higher degrees of clinical skill and experience, in addition to considerably higher laboratory costs.

In general, removable provisional restorations may be more straightforward to fabricate, often at a lower laboratory cost. For clinicians, removable restorations may also be easier to deliver and adjust. Removable prostheses can be borne by the tooth and/or soft tissue. Tissue-borne removable prostheses will likely be associated with increased and intermittent loading or pressure on the grafted or implant sites during the healing process. This may jeopardize the optimal result of augmentation or implant procedures. Further, poorly designed prostheses may have a negative impact on the final soft tissue result. Careful attention is therefore required with regard to fit and adaptation of removable prostheses.

Fixed Provisional Options

Phase I provisional restorations, utilized between tooth extraction and implant placement, are an important treatment step (Chee 2001; Priest 2006; Santosa 2007). They are used primarily to satisfy the patient's masticatory and esthetic requirements. In addition, they maintain stability both within the dental arch, and with the opposing teeth. Provisional restorations used at this stage can, however, also be utilized to contour soft tissue and direct healing so as to improve the site for implant placement, and increase the likelihood of an optimal outcome.

The options for phase I provisional restorations include a cast metal or fiber-reinforced resin-bonded fixed prosthesis (RBFP) or a partial fixed prosthesis.

Cast Metal or Fiber-Reinforced Resin-Bonded Fixed Prostheses

A RBFP with or without an ovate pontic may be used as a provisional or interim restoration if sufficient interocclusal space is available. Such space is needed both for occlusion and to contour the soft tissue prior to implant placement and/or loading. A RBFP offers the advantages of a fixed prosthesis – including superior patient comfort and control of pressure to adjacent tissues with minimal interference at the implant or graft site. Resin-bonded interim prostheses should only be in contact with small areas of etched enamel for retention on adjacent teeth. Pontic options include acrylic or composite resin denture teeth, metal-ceramic pontics (with cast metal frameworks), ceramic denture teeth or extracted crowns, and extracted natural teeth (Figure 7.1).

Each of these options can be modified to incorporate a cast metal or polyethylene ribbon designed as both reinforcement and as the prosthesis retainer. The laboratory costs may be substantial, most notably for a metal-ceramic RBFP (Figure 7.2).

The cost of a fiber-reinforced RBFP is relatively low. The procedure is also less complicated for both the technician and clinician.

Resin-bonded fixed provisional restorations are not recommended when multiple surgical procedures (extraction, ridge augmentation, implant placement, second stage surgery) are anticipated. Constant removal and repositioning may be detrimental to both the adjacent teeth and the provisional restoration. Fiber-reinforced options are, for the most part, not reusable subsequent to removal.

Partial Fixed Prostheses

In situations where full coverage restorations are planned for teeth adjacent to the implant site, these teeth can be used to retain and support provisional fixed restorations (Figure 7.3).

This option can provide a convenient and predictable provisional solution. The provisional restorations can be fabricated chairside or in a dental laboratory, and may be contoured to encourage tissue shape and healing. Although most prostheses of this type are fabricated using auto-polymerizing acrylic resin or composite, the dental laboratory may also process a more durable prosthesis with customized texture and shade using a heat-polymerizing material. This may provide a superior esthetic and functional outcome, although at a higher cost.

Provisional fixed prostheses can be fabricated prior to extraction and/or implant placement via the indirect method, so they are ready in time for the surgical procedure. This can make the treatment phase easier for the patient to tolerate. Pontic modification can also be done throughout the healing and tissue maturation period by adding or subtracting resin material from the tissue contact areas. As with alternative fixed provisional options, controlled pressure can be applied on the implant site to achieve optimal tissue contours.

Removable Provisional Options

Vacuum-Formed Removable Retainer Supporting an Ovate Pontic

A vacuum-formed removable retainer supporting an ovate pontic (Essix retainer) can be an effective and satisfying provisional restoration. Interocclusal space is often restricted and difficult to achieve before soft or hard tissue augmentation procedures. Provisional options other than the Essix retainer can be challenging to use. An Essix retainer is usually easy to fabricate, is relatively inexpensive, and can be a convenient option prior to making a longer lasting provisional prosthesis. A denture tooth, or extracted tooth, can be modified to fit the pontic site and to esthetically match the adjacent dentition. The tissue contact areas at the pontic site can be adjusted to an ovate shape in order to achieve optimal soft tissue contours. It can also be modified to be completely free of tissue contact.

A vacuum-formed appliance is tooth retained and supported, however it is still considered to be a removable prosthesis. Although it may provide the advantage of applying controlled pressure at the implant site, there are the usual disadvantages of a removable prosthesis. Patient compliance in wearing the prosthesis in order to continually contour the soft tissue at the implant site is important. Removable provisional options may be occlusally uncomfortable. They are, however, resistant to catastrophic fracture and are often readily accepted.

Interim Removable Partial Dental Prosthesis

Interim removable prostheses are commonly used as they are relatively inexpensive and easy to fabricate (Figure 7.4). For patients who require multiple surgical procedures, interim removable prostheses are also readily modified and adjusted. Acrylic resin can be added and subtracted to accommodate changes to the implant site. Additional denture teeth can be added to an existing prosthesis at minimal cost and little added discomfort to the patient.

Removable provisional prostheses are, however, associated with several shortcomings. For many patients, the discomfort of wearing a removable prosthesis with added bulk can be problematic. These

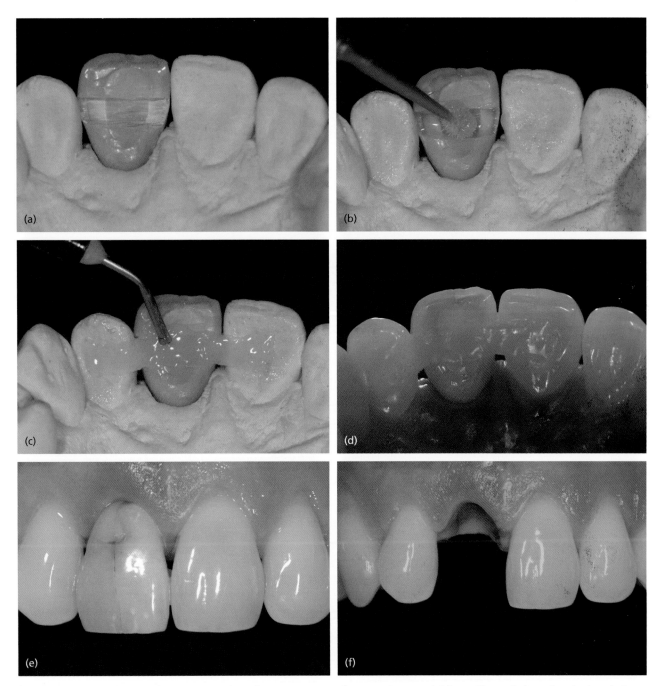

Figure 7.1 Clinical case where extracted tooth no. 8 was used as pontic material for a fiber-reinforced resin-bonded prosthesis prior to implant loading. (a) The study cast and extracted tooth were modified to create a convex pontic shape and the lingual aspect of the extracted tooth was prepared to accommodate the reinforcement bondable fiber. (b) The prepared tooth surface was acid etched using 37% phosphoric acid, and thoroughly rinsed, dried, and treated with a bonding agent; the surfaces of the retainer teeth were applied with separating medium. (c) A light-polymerizing flowable composite was used to connect the reinforcement fibers with the pontic material and to impregnate these fibers for retainer wing fabrication. (d, e) The laboratory-fabricated prosthesis was bonded in place: (d) occlusal view and (e) facial view. (f) Facial soft tissue profile after 3 months of soft tissue development prior to implant loading.

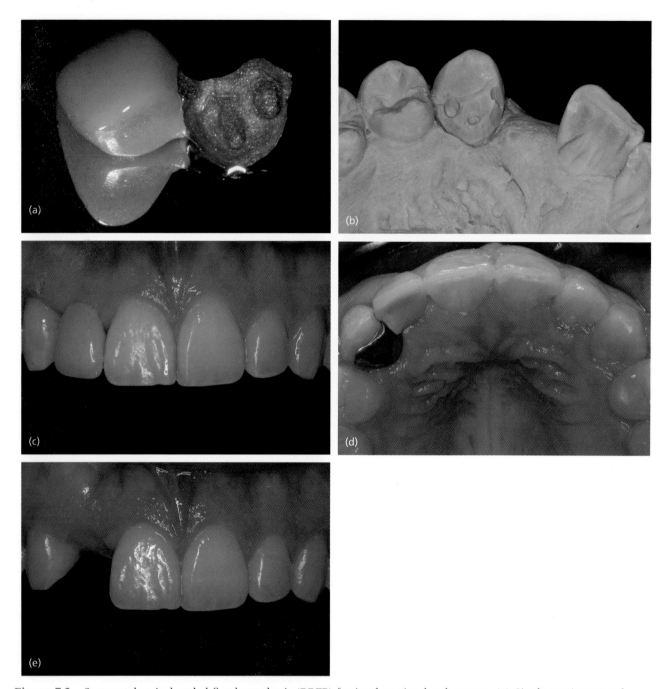

Figure 7.2   Cast metal resin-bonded fixed prosthesis (RBFP) for implant site development. (a) Single-retainer metal-ceramic RBFP. (b) Definitive cast demonstrating abutment teeth preparation at site no. 6 for the RBFP retainer. (c, d) RBFP in situ for implant site development prior to implant placement: (c) facial view and (d) occlusal view. (e) Soft tissue profile contoured by the RBFP pontic at site no. 10.

prostheses may also interfere with speech, consequently reducing patient compliance. Passivity of fit may also present concerns, most notably uncontrolled or undesirable pressure on the soft tissue.

An interim partial prosthesis also requires sufficient interocclusal space to maintain adequate strength of the prosthesis, in addition to the incorporation of components designed to improve stability and support. For patients with minimal space between opposing dentitions, thin connector areas are prone to fracture. The need for repeated repair is frustrating for both the patient and the clinician. Although it is possible to develop the soft tissue profile using an ovate pontic on the interim removable prosthesis, a fixed prosthesis with controlled vertical pressure is preferred.

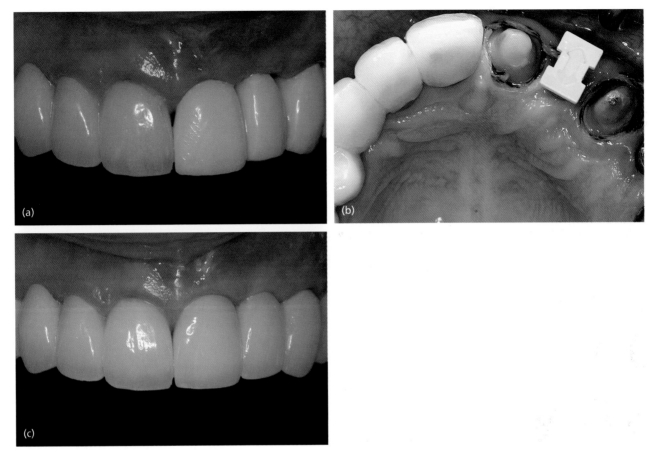

Figure 7.3 (a) Provisional fixed partial denture (site nos 9, 10, and 11) fabricated with auto-polymerizing acrylic resin inserted with the pontic at the no. 10 area for implant site development after tissue augmentation. (b) Close tray fixture-level impression technique used for a definitive impression. (c) Definitive zirconia-ceramic single-unit restorations at nos 9, 10, and 11. A narrow-diameter (3.3 mm) implant was used with a prefabricated titanium abutment.

CONTOURING THE SOFT TISSUE WITH PROVISIONAL AND CUSTOM IMPRESSIONS

Traditionally, conservative loading guidelines have been recommended in implant treatment protocols – often as long as 3–6 months. With improved implant morphology and surface design, including enhanced hydrophilicity and chemical reactivity, accelerated loading protocols (between 6 and 8 weeks for most implants) can be used. Implant survivial has not been found to be affected (Grütter and Belser 2009).

The maturation and stabilization of peri-implant soft tissue around provisional restorations requires additional time to allow for bone healing. Where soft tissue healing occurs alongside the bone healing (if the restoration is immediately placed and loaded), it is less predictable from the esthetic perspective. Recessions of up to 1 mm are common (Oates et al. 2002). For this reason it is most commonly recommended in the esthetic zone to load implants a minimum of 6–8 weeks subsequent to their placement, irrespective of the placement protocol.

The cylindrical cervical profiles of prefabricated healing abutments (Figure 7.5a) differ greatly in size and shape from the desired, somewhat triangular, profile of teeth and esthetic anterior definitive restorations (Figure 7.5b).

In addition, the emergence profile of implant-based provisional restorations often requires contour modification during the healing process to improve or reduce tissue support. In the esthetic zone, recontouring of provisional restorations to improve the esthetic tissue response may be critical to the outcome. Interdental papillae in the esthetic zone often form an acute angle or point at their coronal apex when correctly formed. A lack of support for the papillae will often result in the apical migration of the acute tissue point, and the formation of a flat surface. The region above the flat surface (which should ideally be occupied by the papillae) is an isosceles triangular shape devoid of tissue. This has become known as the "black triangle or space." The papillae can be encouraged to reoccupy the region.

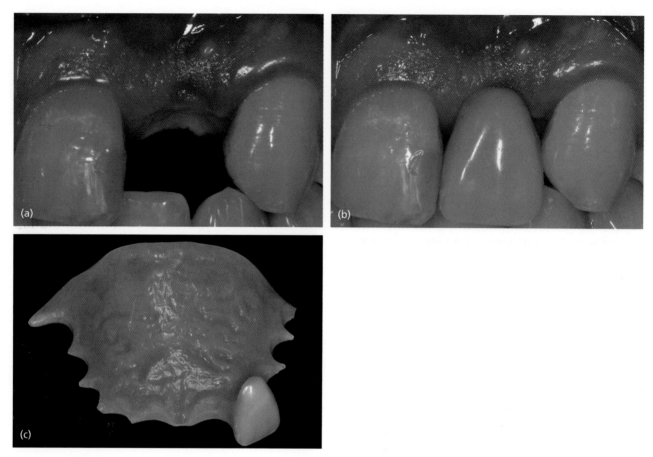

Figure 7.4   (a) Soft tissue contoured by the ovate-shaped pontic with an interim removable partial denture. (b) Interim removable partial denture in situ. (c) Design of the interim removable partial denture.

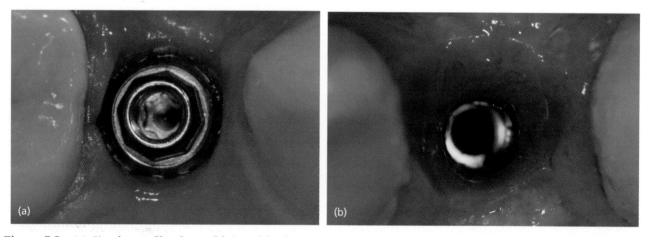

Figure 7.5   (a) Circular profile of a prefabricated healing abutment. (b) Emergence profile on the peri-implant soft tissue after tissue contouring with a provisional restoration.

Provisional restorations overcontoured in the interdental areas bring the emerging surfaces of the adjacent teeth into proximity too quickly. The result is interdental closure as a result of oversized teeth and too much contact between them. In these areas the papillae are shorter than ideal, and often more obtuse

in angulation. In these circumstances, material can be carefully removed from the provisional restoration to facilitate improved contours. It is important to note that complications of this type are often associated with implants and components that are too large for the particular esthetic site. Implants with improved

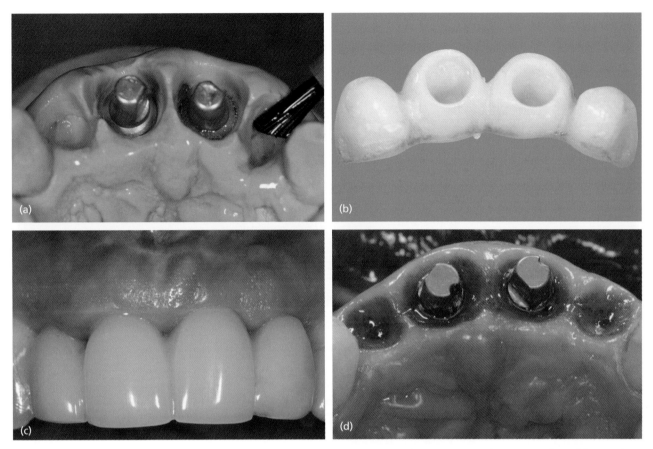

Figure 7.6 Cement-retained provisional restoration fabricated with auto-polymerizing acrylic resin and prefabricated implant abutments. (a) The abutment-level impression technique was used to obtain the master cast. The pontic sites at no. 7 and no. 10, along with peri-implant areas at no. 8 and no. 9, were contoured on the cast for ideal soft tissue development. Separating medium was applied prior to the provisional restoration fabrication. (b) Intaglio surface of the restoration with the desired peri-implant emergence profile and convex-shaped pontics. (c) Provisional restoration in situ. (d) Peri-implant soft tissue profile contoured with the provisional restoration after 3 months.

physical properties and morphology alleviate some of these issues.

Prefabricated, contoured implant abutments for a definitive prosthesis may improve the emergence profile, but they cannot manage all clinical conditions. In order to optimize esthetic outcomes, it is essential, for most sites, to place a provisional restoration onto the implant subsequent to healing. It should then be customized to facilitate the maturation and stabilization of peri-implant soft tissues. These procedures are the most predictable and practical method of insuring a natural esthetic soft tissue profile (Martin et al. 2007).

Cement-retained Provisional Restorations

Prefabricated abutments designed for cemented definitive restorations may be used to retain provisional restorations (Hebel and Gajjar 1997; Michalakis et al. 2003; Chee and Jivraj 2006a, 2006b; Lee et al. 2010). This method of fabrication should use prefabricated provisional copings for the cemented restorations to minimize issues relating to poor fit. These abutments may be torqued to less than the manufacturer's recommendation (and remain in place during the provisional phase). Later they can be removed with no detrimental influence on the implant (Figure 7.6).

The most significant challenge of this technique is the limited access for the removal of excess cement. The peri-implant tissues in the esthetic zone are often deeply scalloped, making predictable excess removal impossible. The excess residual cement often leads to peri-implant inflammation, which may result in bone loss and subsequent soft tissue complications. Great caution needs to be exercised during the cementation procedures.

A meso abutment or modified prefabricated abutment can be used to individualize the cement margin for implant-retained provisional restorations. Modified

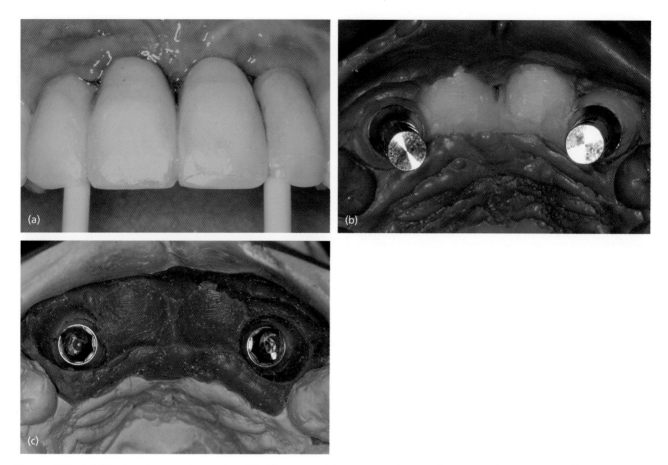

Figure 7.7   (a) Plastic tubes can be used as blocking material to prevent impression material getting into the screw access. The open tray technique can be used for implant fixture impressions. (b) Implant fixture analogs attached to the provisional restoration prior to making the cast. (c) Peri-implant soft tissue profile and pontic profile transferred from the provisional restoration to the soft tissue cast.

abutments can bring cement margins circumferentially to within 1 or 2 mm of the free gingival margins. This improves the likelihood of effective removal. This is often feasible for clinicians who are able to use conventional fabrication methods incorporating a vacuum-formed matrix or polycarbonate crown.

Screw-retained Provisional Restorations

There are several advantages offered by screw-retained provisional restorations on dental implants (Hebel and Gajjar 1997; Michalakis et al. 2003; Chee and Jivraj 2006b; Lee et al. 2010). First, the possibility of residual cement is completely eliminated. Second, screw-retained provisional restorations can be positioned more predictably as the screw pulls the provisional restoration against the tissue. The machined abutment also fits more accurately to the implant – increasing the quality of the tissue response.

Screw-retained provisional restorations can be used directly as an impression coping to transfer the peri-

implant soft tissue profile (Figure 7.7). The peri-implant soft tissues often require slow and sequenced expansion during the initial insertion of the provisional restoration (Figure 7.8). This is due to the restoration's natural emergence profile as compared with that of the healing abutment.

Figure 7.9 illustrates the direct (chairside) fabrication technique for screw-retained provisional restorations.

Customized Impression Technique

Provisional restorations should be monitored for a minimum of 4 weeks, and for as long as 3 months, to facilitate the maturation and stability of the peri-implant soft tissues. Any modifications made to the provisional form during this time period may increase the period required for observation. This process should be considered mandatory in the esthetic zone. Compared with the root of a natural tooth, dental implants often exhibit a smaller diameter along their cylindrical shape.

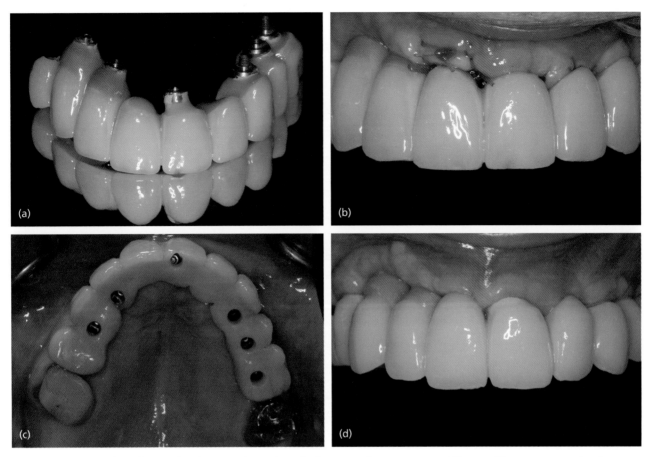

Figure 7.8 (a) Implant fixture-level impression taken during second-stage surgery. The maxillary screw-retained provisional restoration was fabricated in the dental laboratory using the indirect technique. (b, c) Provisional restorations in situ: (b) facial view and (c) occlusal view. (d) Definitive metal-ceramic restorations.

In most anterior esthetic sites, the sulcus around implant-based restorations can vary in depth and often exceeds 5 mm. Once the desired peri-implant soft tissue profile has been achieved with the provisional restoration, an accurate cast of the emergence profile should be made (Chee and Jivraj 2006a; Hämmerle and Jung 2007). A customized impression coping that duplicates the new sulcus form can be made with a two-stage process: the open tray technique (Figure 7.10) and closed tray technique (Figure 7.11).

DIFFERENT DESIGNS OF FINAL CROWNS SUPPORTED BY CUSTOM AND STOCK ABUTMENTS

The esthetic outcome of implant restorations is dependent largely on rigorous pre-treatment planning and careful patient selection. The management of anatomic limitations, and skillful execution of the surgical and restorative phases, is critical. For most treatment teams, using surgical templates developed from the planning and diagnostic phases is a critical phase, insuring that implants can be positioned in the most optimal locations.

Custom abutments increase the cost of the procedure for the patient and the complexity of fabrication for the dental technician. The quality of the definitive restoration may be enhanced, however, by the lack of a screw access hole (Hebel and Gajjar 1997; Michalakis et al. 2003; Chee and Jivraj 2006b; Lee et al. 2010) (see Chapter 2).

Screw-retained Prostheses

The use of screw-retained restorations is often limited by the trajectory of the implant in the anterior maxilla. Direct palatal screw access is needed and this may result in part of the implant lying outside the bone available, either coronally or at the depth of the vestibule. If the implant trajectory, as a result of surgical or anatomic limitations, results in the screw access being in the esthetic areas (facial or incisal areas), then angled or transversal screw-retained abutments (Figure 7.12) may be considered. It is also possible to use a

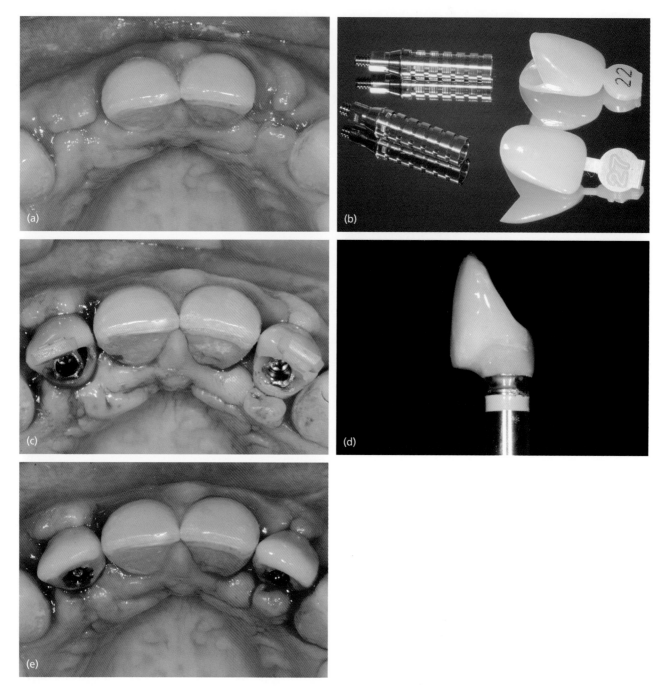

Figure 7.9 (a) Occlusal view of implant sites no. 7 and no. 10 prior to second-stage surgery. (b) Titanium temporary cylinders and polycarbonate crowns. (c) The temporary cylinders were trimmed and polycarbonate crowns adjusted to enclose the temporary cylinders. Auto-polymerizing acrylic resin was used to connect them. (d) Profile of a provisional restoration completed with auto-polymerizing acrylic resin in the laboratory. (e) Complete screw-retained provisional restorations.

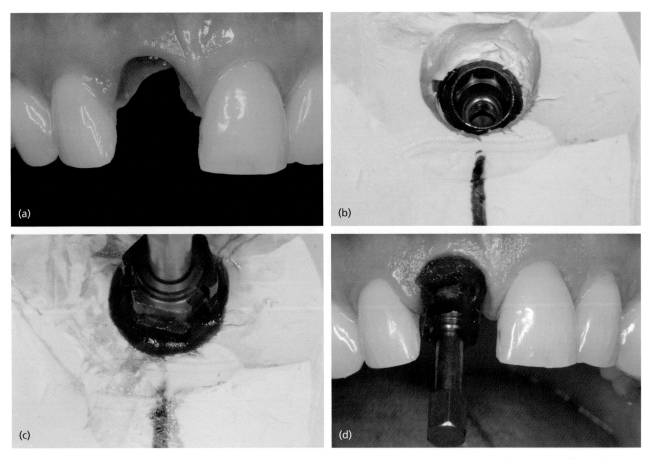

Figure 7.10 Customized impression coping using the open tray technique. (a) Peri-implant soft tissue profile to be transferred. (b) The provisional restoration was removed from the implant and attached to the implant analog and then placed in a plastic cup. Polyvinyl siloxane bite registration material was secreted around the assembly. The vertical mark indicates the facial aspect of the provisional restoration so the impression coping could be correctly orientated. Once the material has set, the provisional restoration was removed. (c) A flowable resin (GC pattern resin, GC America) was used to customize the impression coping with the emergence profile. (d) Facial view of a customized open tray impression coping.

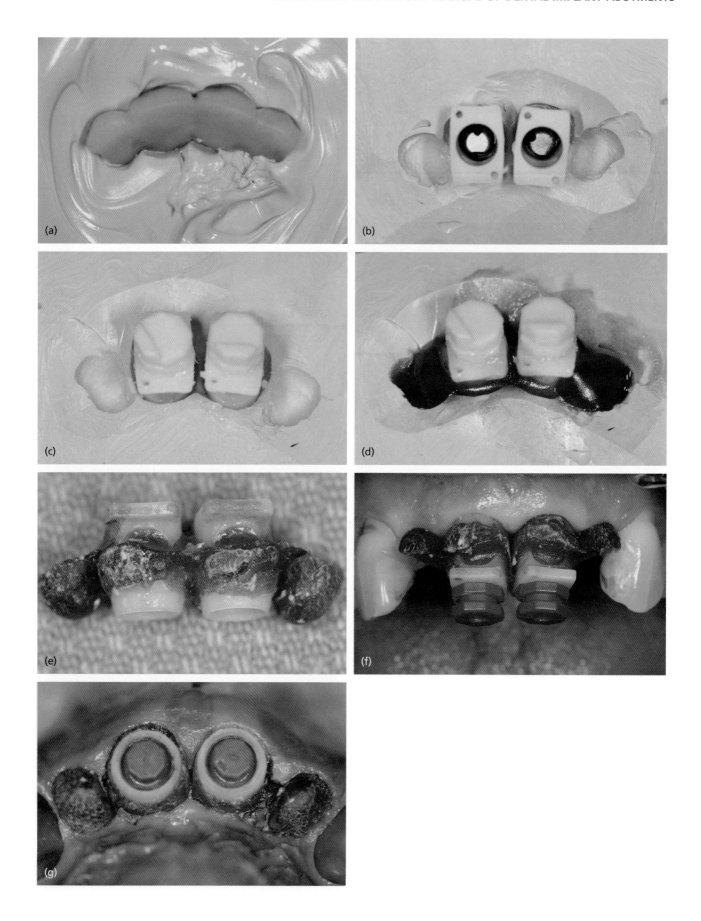

screw-retained custom abutment at the depth of the implant designed to support a cemented restoration.

It can be difficult to achieve an ideal placement for screw-retained implant restorations in the esthetic zone. Esthetic zone (anterior maxillary) teeth are often limited in their orofacial dimension, resulting in a restricted space for screw access. However, if the treatment goal is to use a screw-retained implant restoration, this is often possible with careful pre-treatment planning and execution (Figure 7.13).

Planning with diagnostic wax-ups as the blueprint for the definitive restoration and well-constructed and stable surgical templates are the first prerequisites.

Cement-retained Protheses

For cement-retained restorations with deep margins, it is a significant challenge to access and remove all the residual cement. If cement is left behind then peri-implant soft tissue inflammation and bone loss can occur and cause severe biologic complications. It is therefore essential to confirm complete residual cement removal at the time of crown cementation. Many clinical techniques have been proposed to facilitate this, such as placing petroleum jelly on the outer surface of the crown to reduce the adherence of residual cement, the use of curettes to carefully scale around the crown after cementation, and the meticulous use of dental floss to clean the interproximal areas or the intaglio surfaces underneath the pontics.

However, it is even more important to achieve the correct emergence profile of the abutments and crowns and to place the restorative margin properly.

Abutments for cement-retained implant restorations can be simply categorized as either stock or custom abutments. Stock abutments are fabricated by implant manufacturers and the marginal placement and emergency profile of the abutment are usually made to average dimensions. There are limited choices available that will usually accommodate only the most common clinical situations. The margins and profiles on stock abutments are usually circular with little correlation to the mucosal levels. Even with the new anatomic abutments (abutments with a scalloped margin following the profile and level of the gingival crest), the choice of stock abutments is usually limited. Potential problems of residual cement and difficult management of soft tissues can be expected with their use (Figure 7.14).

Implants are often placed 3 mm or more below the facial soft tissue margin to insure the optimal esthetic outcome. However, with the design of stock abutments, this often leads to a deep interproximal margin of up to 5–6 mm subgingivally. Deep margins can lead to difficulties in removing residual cement, and in maintaining the soft tissue profile after restoration removal. The use of stock abutments should be used only when there is minimal scalloping of the mucosal margins and cement margins can be kept within 2–3 mm of the gingival margin to facilitate cement removal (Figures 7.15 and 7.16).

When the principles of proper margin location placement and appropriate profile design to support the soft tissues are followed, most of the problems of cementation with stock abutments can be overcome.

Custom abutments can be either waxed and cast onto machined cylinders (Figures 7.17 and 7.18) or machined from titanium or zirconia using CAD (e.g. Biomet 3i Encode®, Nobel Biocare Procera®, Zimmer Dental, Atlantis Components, Straumann CARES®), or copied from a waxed form (Nobel Biocare Procera).

Customized metal-ceramic or zirconia abutments can increase the pink esthetics of a definitive restoration in a patient with a thin tissue biotype.

Figure 7.11 Customized impression coping using the close tray technique (same clinical case as in Figure 7.10). (a) A cement-retained provisional restoration was supported on a prefabricated abutment which was removed and attached to the corresponding implant abutment analog. The assembly was then embedded in a plastic cup with polyvinyl siloxane bite registration material. (b) Once the polyvinyl siloxane material set, the provisional restoration was removed. Impression caps were placed on the implant abutment analog. (c) Positioning cylinder (yellow) designed for the corresponding prefabricated abutment which was then attached to the impression cap (white). (d) A flowable resin (GC pattern resin, GC America) was used to customize the impression coping with the emergence and pontic profile. (e) The customized impression cap captured the peri-implant soft tissue and pontic profile. (f) The customized impression cap and positioning cylinder were used for the implant-level impression. (g) Final impression with customized impression cap and positioning cylinder in place.

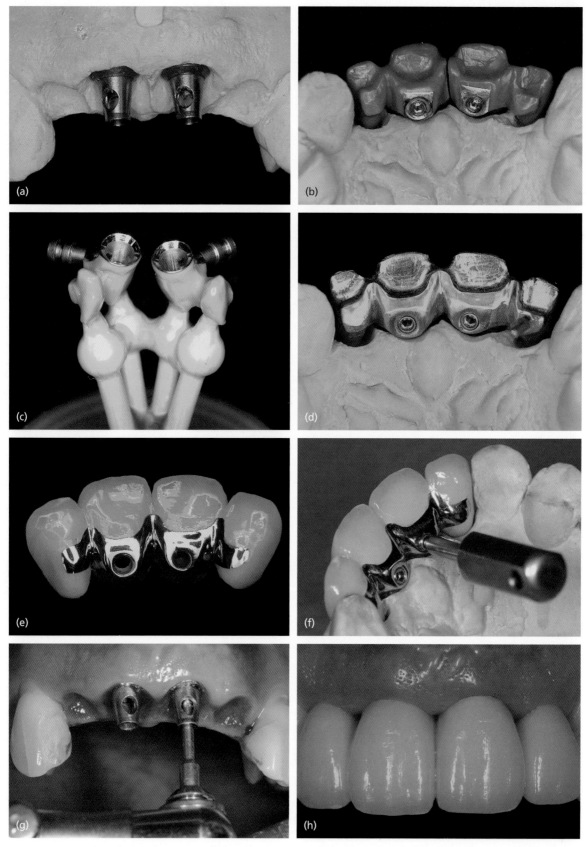

Figure 7.12 Screw-retained prosthesis with a transversal screw (TS). This allowed a lingual path of insertion for the restoration fixation screw (same clinical case as in Figure 7.11). (a) TS abutments were fitted to the master cast. Note the peri-implant soft tissue and pontic were transferred onto the master cast with customized impression coping. (b) TS gold copings were seated on the TS abutments and modified with wax. (c) The completed wax patterns were invested and selected alloy used for casting. (d) Completed metal framework ready for subsequent porcelain application. (e) Completed definitive metal-ceramic restorations. (f) Lingual set screws and TS screwdriver used to secure the restorations onto the TS abutments. (g) At the insertion appointment, the TS abutments were torqued in the implants. The restorations were then inserted in place with lingual set screws and a TS screwdriver. (h) Facial view of the definitive TS restorations.

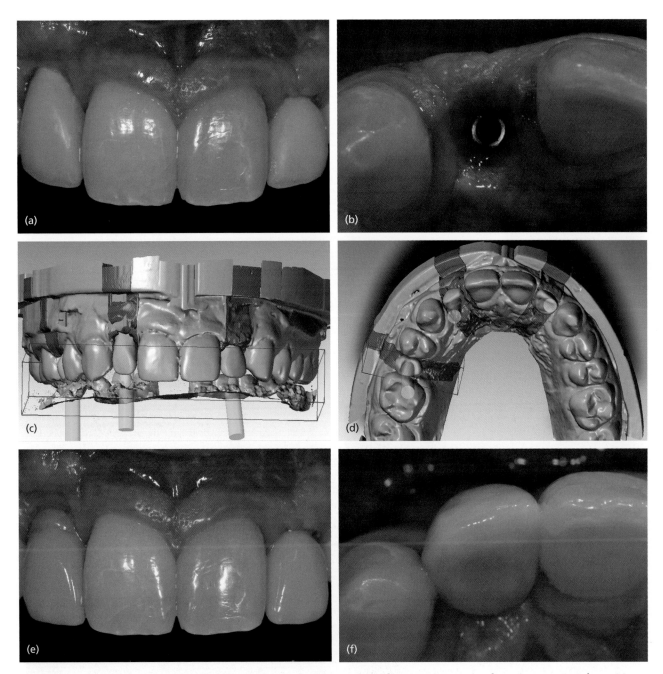

Figure 7.13 One-piece zirconia screw-retained crowns. (a) Provisional restorations at implant sites no. 7 and no. 10. (b) Occlusal view of the soft tissue profile at implant site no. 10 after 3 months of provisionalization. (c, d) Screenshots of CAD/CAM zirconia substructure design where the green tubes illustrate the screw access trajectories: (c) frontal view and (d) occlusal view. (e) Screw-retained zirconia-ceramic restorations were inserted. The no. 7 restoration had pink porcelain to compensate for a soft tissue defect. (f) Occlusal view of the restoration at site no. 10. The screw access was sealed with a cotton pellet and light-polymerizing composite.

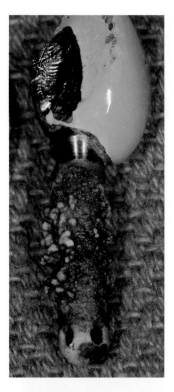

Figure 7.14   Failed implant with residual cement.

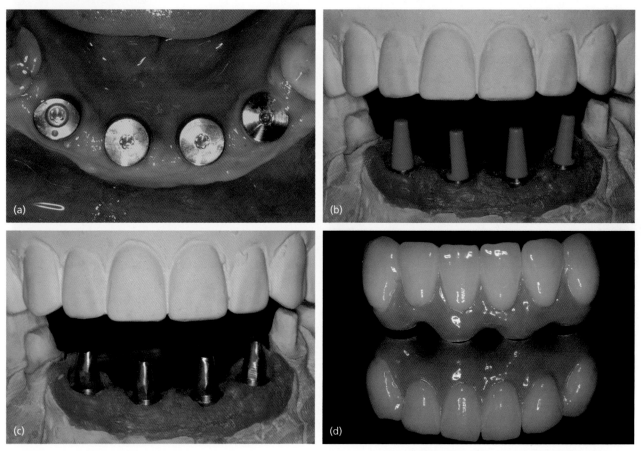

Figure 7.15   Cement-retained implant restoration with stock abutments where there was minimal scalloping of the mucosal margins and the cement margins were within 2mm of the gingival margin. (a) Anterior mandibular implants were integrated. (b) Planning abutments were used to choose the prefabricated abutments. (c) Straight prefabricated titanium cementable abutments were chosen and minor adjustments were made to achieve the desired path of insertion. (d) Definitive cement-retained metal-ceramic fixed partial implants. The interproximal areas were designed with space for the ease of hygiene access.

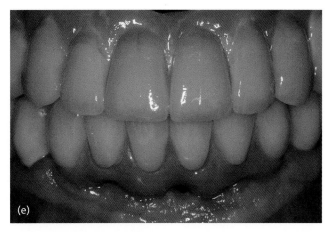

Figure 7.15 (*Continued*) (e) Frontal view of the maxillary and mandibular definitive metal-ceramic restorations.

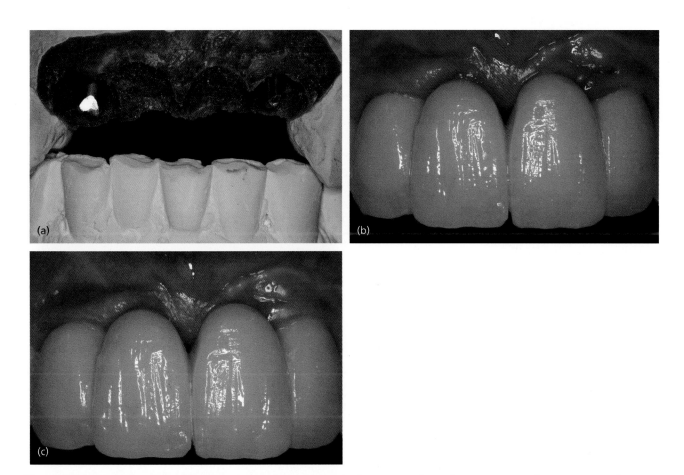

Figure 7.16 Cement-retained implant restoration with stock abutments where the cement margins were more than 2–3 mm from the gingival margin. (a) Deeply placed implants with stock abutments for cement-retained restorations. (b) Sinus tracts developed at 1 month after the crown was fitted; the residual cement was removed carefully. (c) Two-year follow-up with healthy peri-implant soft tissue.

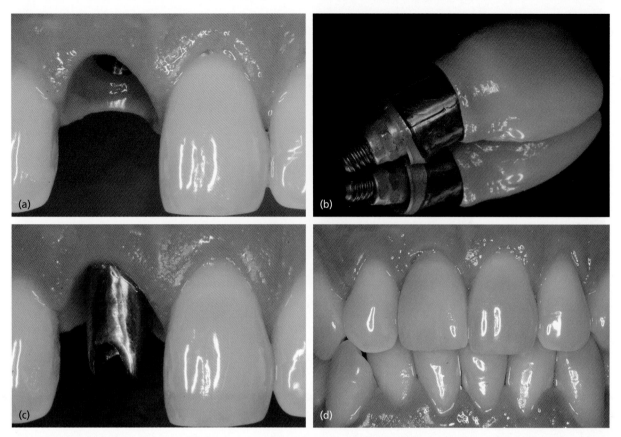

Figure 7.17 Cement-retained restoration with customized cementable metal abutment (same clinical case as in Figure 7.1). (a) Soft tissue profile after 3 months of development with an implant-retained provisional restoration. (b) Customized cementable metal abutment with a definitive metal-ceramic restoration. (c) Customized cementable metal abutment in situ. (d) Definitve metal-ceramic restoration.

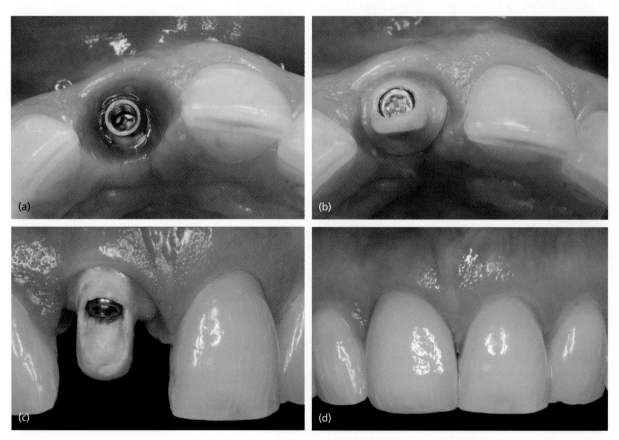

Figure 7.18 Cement-retained restoration with customized metal-ceramic abutment (same clinical case as in Figure 7.10). (a) Soft tissue profile after 3 months of soft tissue development with an implant-retained provisional restoration. (b, c) Customized cementable metal-ceramic abutment in situ: (c) occlusal view and (d) facial view. (d) Definitve metal-ceramic restoration.

REFERENCES AND ADDITIONAL READING

Buser, D., Martin, W., & Belser, U.C. (2004). Optimizing esthetics for implant restorations in the anterior maxilla: anatomic and surgical considerations. *International Journal of Oral and Maxillofacial Implants,* 19 (Suppl), S43–61.

Chee, W. (2001). Provisional restorations in soft tissue management around dental implants. *Periodontology 2000,* 27, 139–147.

Chee, W. & Jivraj, S. (2006a). Impression techniques for implant dentistry. *British Dental Journal,* 201, 429–432.

Chee, W. & Jivraj, S. (2006b). Screw versus cemented implant supported restorations. *British Dental Journal,* 201, 501–507.

Hämmerle, C. & Jung, R. (2007). Prosthetic management of implants in the esthetic zone: general principles and scientific documentation. In *ITI Treatment Guide, I: Implant Therapy in the Esthetic Zone: Single Tooth Replacements,* ed. Buser, D., Belser, U., & Wismeijer, D. Berlin: Quintessence Publishing, 38–48.

Hebel, K.S. & Gajjar, R.C. (1997). Cement-retained versus screw-retained implant restorations: achieving optimal occlusion and esthetics in implant dentistry. *Journal of Prosthetic Dentistry,* 77, 28–35.

Higginbottom, F., Belser, U., Jones, J.D., & Keith, S.E. (2004). Prosthetic management of implants in the esthetic zone. *International Journal of Oral and Maxillofacial Implants,* 19(Suppl), S62–72.

Grütter, L. & Belser, U.C. (2009). Implant loading protocols for the partially edentulous esthetic zone. *International Journal of Oral and Maxillofacial Implants,* 24(Suppl), S169–179.

Lee, A., Okayasu, K., & Wang, H.L. (2010). Screw- versus cement-retained implant restorations: current concepts. *Implant Dentistry,* 19, 8–15.

Martin, W.C., Morton, D., & Buser, D. (2007). Pre-operative analysis and prosthetic treatment planning in esthetic implant dentistry. In *ITI Treatment Guide, I: Implant Therapy in the Esthetic Zone: Single Tooth Replacements,* ed. Buser, D., Belser, U., & Wismeijer, D. Chicago: Quintessence Publishing, 9–24.

Michalakis, K.X., Hirayama, H., & Garefis, P.D. (2003). Cement-retained versus screw-retained implant restorations: a critical review. *International Journal of Oral and Maxillofacial Implants,* 18, 719–728.

Oates, T.W., West, J., Jones, J., Kaiser, D., & Cochran, D.L. (2002). Long-term changes in soft tissue height on the facial surface of dental implants. *Implant Dentistry,* 11, 272–279.

Priest, G. (2006). Esthetic potential of single-implant provisional restorations: selection criteria of available alternatives. *Journal of Esthetic and Restorative Dentistry,* 18, 326–338.

Santosa, R.E. (2007). Provisional restoration options in implant dentistry. *Australian Dental Journal,* 52, 234–242.

8

Instrumentation for Abutment Modification and Guidelines for their Use

Hamid R. Shafie

Washington Hospital Center, Department of Oral and Maxillofacial Surgery, Washington, DC; and American Institute of Implant Dentistry, Washington, DC

INTRODUCTION

Titanium and zirconia abutments are currently the most commonly used prosthetic parts used to support the final prosthesis. Whether a clinician or laboratory technician uses a stock abutment or a CAD/CAM-generated abutment, it is sometimes necessary to adjust the abutment to idealize the contour, emergence profile, and location of finish line.

Adjusting implant abutments requires specific rotary instruments. When these are being used it is important to follow the instructions for use and procedure manual. This prevents any damage to the implant abutment, especially zirconia.

Zirconia is very reliable and durable, yet difficult to work on. The grinding and adjusting of zirconia abutments constitutes a real challenge for dentists and dental technicians. Because zirconia is so hard, it is important to use instruments that have particularly strongly bonded diamond grains and a higher operating life than usual.

In this chapter adjustment sequences for titanium and zirconia abutments will be discussed.

EXTRA-ORAL ADJUSTMENT TECHNIQUES FOR A TITANIUM ABUTMENT

The Vitality Laboratory rotary instruments kit for titanium abutment adjustment has been designed for adjusting titanium abutments (Figure 8.1). Instruments should be mounted on an electric or air-driven straight handpiece with an rpm (revolutions per minute) adjustment feature. To maximize the performance of these instruments, your handpiece should be capable of providing a range of 5000–50,000 rpm. No irrigation or coolant is required for use.

Cutting Instruments

Vitality cutting instruments are made of highly compressed, fine grain carbide (Figure 8.2). Each instrument is application specific.

- *Black:* This should be used for major gross reduction of the incisal and lingual surfaces of a titanium abutment. This instrument helps in the rapid

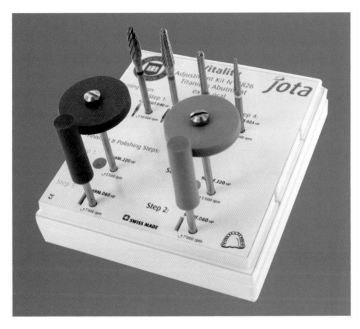

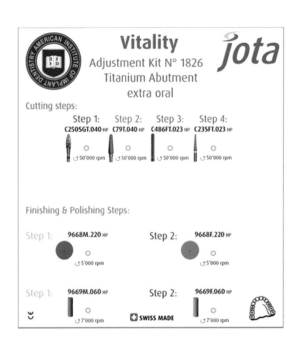

Figure 8.1   Vitality rotary instrument kit for titanium abutments.

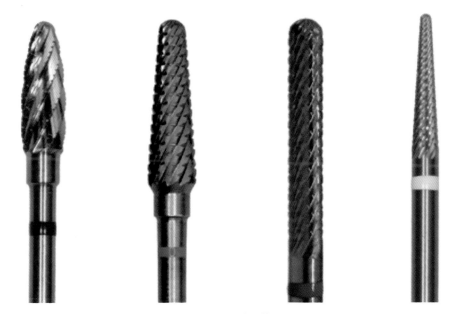

Figure 8.2   Titanium cutting instruments: black, blue, red, and yellow.

reduction of metal volume. It should not be used for defined reduction.

- *Blue:* This should be used for more defined reductions of the labial, lingual, mesial, and distal surfaces.
- *Red:* This should be used to define a chamfer finish line.
- *Yellow:* This should be used to finalize the taper angle between the mesial and distal surfaces, as well as reducing any scratches left by the other instruments.

Note: All of these instruments should be used at 50,000 rpm. These instruments will not be as effective with other metals due to the specific angulations of the blades. They should be replaced after 10 abutment adjustments.

Finishing and Polishing Instruments

The silicone-based polishing instruments make up a two-step polishing system (Figure 8.3) using the two types of rubbers.

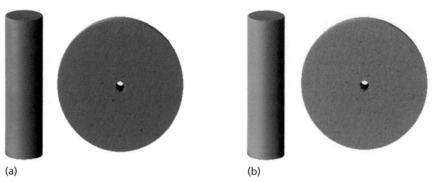

Figure 8.3   Silicone rubbers for polishing the surface of titanium abutments: (a) dark blue pre-polisher and (b) light blue fine polisher.

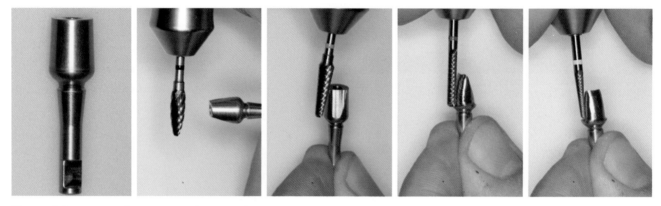

Figure 8.4   Gross reduction steps for a titanium abutment.

- *Dark blue pre-polisher:* This reduces and smoothes all the scratches left behind during the cutting step.
- *Light blue fine polisher:* This polishes the surface of the titanium abutment to a high lustre.

These hard polishers have excellent removal capabilities for commercially pure titanium and titanium alloys. The unique combination of abrasive particles and specifically matched synthetic rubber bonding results in an excellent removal rate with reduced heat. Because of their unique composition, they minimize heat development during the polishing process.

Note: To maximize performance of these instruments, they should be used at between 5000 and 7000 rpm.

Adjustment Steps for a Prefabricated Titanium Abutment

Gross Reduction

Step 1. Mark the labial or lingual surface of the abutment before starting gross reduction. If you are adjusting a solid abutment, with more than 2 mm titanium thickness, use the black carbide to reduce the height and the lingual surface (Figure 8.4). If

the abutment has thin walls, skip the black carbide and start with the blue one.

Step 2. The blue carbide should be used to define the labial surface as well as performing less aggressive reduction of the lingual surface. For gross reduction of interproximal surfaces using a thick titanium abutment, use the blue bur.

Step 3. Use the red carbide to create a defined chamfer finish.

Step 4. The yellow carbide is used to define the required taper between the interproximal surfaces. This instrument is also used as a finishing instrument to smooth scratches left from the first three steps.

Note: These instruments should be used at 50,000 rpm with light pressure when grinding.

Finishing and Polishing

Step 1. Use the dark blue wheel to remove scratches from the entire abutment surface except for the finish line (Figure 8.5). Use an abrasive stone to sharpen the tip of the dark blue cylinder polisher. Use the tapered tip to remove any scratches or roughness on the finish line.

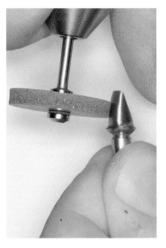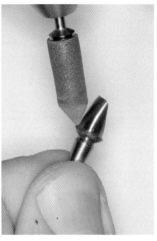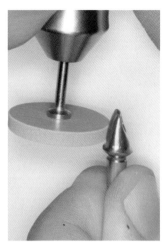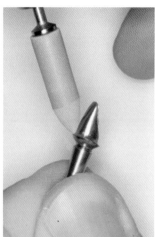

Figure 8.5 Polishing steps for a titanium abutment.

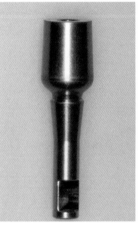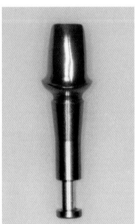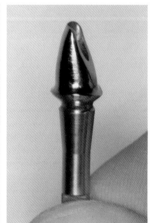

Figure 8.6 Before and after adjustment.

Step 2: Use the light blue wheel to create a luster shine on the entire abutment surface except for the finish line. Use an abrasive stone to sharpen the tip of the light blue cylinder polisher. Use the tapered tip to create a luster shine on the finish line.

Note: These instruments should be used at 5000 rpm. *Do not* apply pressure while using these instruments. It is important to establish a light contact between the instrument and abutment surface to optimize its function. The strokes should be either away from you or toward you to maximize the finishing result (Figure 8.6).

EXTRA-ORAL ADJUSTMENT TECHNIQUES FOR A ZIRCONIA ABUTMENT

The Vitality Laboratory rotary instruments kit for zirconia abutment adjustment has been designed for adjusting ceramic materials such as sintered zirconia abutments (Figure 8.7). These instruments should be mounted on an electric or air-driven straight head-piece with an rpm adjustment feature. To maximize efficiency these instruments have application- and rpm-specific features. For optimal use, the handpiece should be capable of providing a range of 8000–50,000 rpm. No irrigation or coolant is required when these instruments are being used.

Gross Reduction Instruments

- *Green diamond stone wheel:* This sintered diamond stone can be used on all types of ceramic abutments, as well as on titanium (Figure 8.8). However, for optimal performance, it is advised to only use it on ceramic abutments. The green diamond stone wheel should be used for major gross reduction of the incisal and lingual surfaces. It is not recommended for use in creating a defined reduction. Finally, this instrument performs best at 8000 rpm. No irrigation or coolant is required for use.

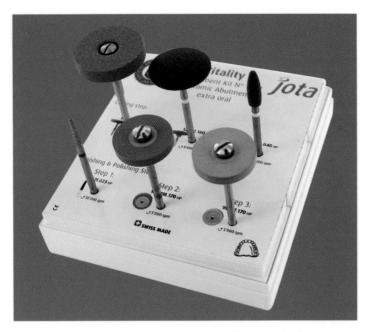

Figure 8.7 Vitality rotary instrument kit for zirconia abutments.

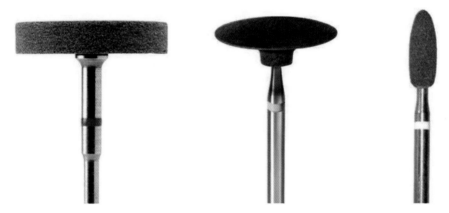

Figure 8.8 Instruments for the gross reduction of zirconia abutments: green diamond stone wheel, black stone wheel, and pear-shaped black stone.

- *Black stone wheel:* This stone is made of silicone carbide. It has been specifically developed for trimming sintered zirconia. It should be used for more defined reduction of labial, lingual, mesial, and distal surfaces. Black stone wheels should be used at 8000 rpm. No irrigation or coolant is required.
- *Pear-shaped black stone:* This instrument is used to finalize the shape of the lingual surface, rounding the sharp edges and reducing the scratches or irregularities on the surface of a zirconia abutment. This instrument should be used at 31,000 rpm. No irrigation or coolant is required.

Finishing and Polishing Instruments

- *Red tapered diamond:* This instrument is made of fine grain diamond and will not chip the abutment edges (Figure 8.9). The red tapered diamond should be used for finalizing the desired tapered walls as well as creating a defined chamfer finish line on the abutment. The recommended rpm is 50,000. No irrigation or coolant is required for its use.
- *Diamond silicone polisher instruments:* This two-step polishing system includes the following types:
  - *Purple pre-polisher:* This removes all the scratches left on the surface of the zirconia abutment after

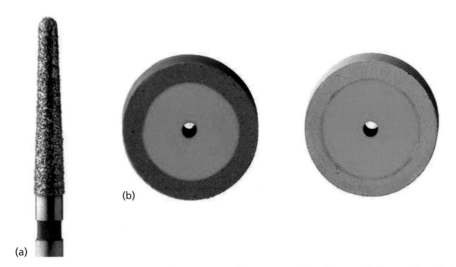

Figure 8.9 Finishing and polishing instruments for zirconia abutments: (a) red tapered diamond and (b) purple and gray polishing system.

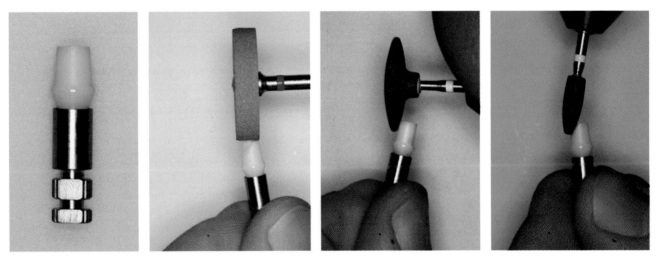

Figure 8.10 Gross reduction steps for a zirconia abutment.

using the gross reduction instruments and red diamond.

— *Gray fine polisher:* This polishes the surface of the zirconia abutment to create a high luster. These are very hard polishers with an excellent removal capability for sintered zirconia abutments. Both of these polishers should be used at 5000 rpm. Because of their unique composition, there will be minimal heat development during the polishing process. No irrigation or coolant is required for use.

Adjustment Steps for a Prefabricated Zirconia Abutment

Gross Reduction

Step 1. Mark the labial or lingual surface on the abutment before starting gross reduction. Use the green diamond stone to reduce the lingual surface as well as the height (Figure 8.10). If an abutment with thin walls is being modified skip the green diamond stone and go straight to the black zirconflex stones.

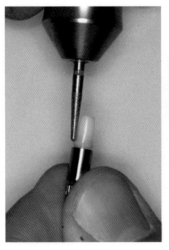 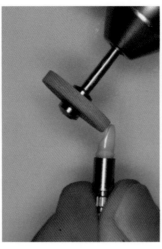 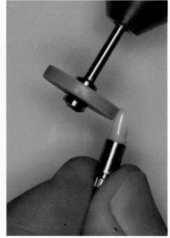 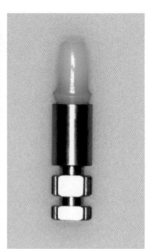

Figure 8.11   Finishing and polishing steps for a zirconia abutment.

Step 2. Use the black stone wheel to define the shape of the labial and interproximal surfaces. The taper between the interproximal walls should also be finalized with this instrument. It provides maximum control for a precise grinding.

Step 3. Use the pear-shaped black stone to finalize the shape of the lingual surface, and to round up the sharp edges. This instrument should be used to remove any remaining scratches or irregularities on any of the surfaces of the abutment.

Note: Always use 8000 rpm for the green stone and black stone wheel. The pear-shaped black stone should be used at 31,000 rpm. Regardless of which stone is being utilized, always apply very light pressure. No coolant or irrigation is needed.

Finishing and Polishing

Step 1. Use the red diamond instrument to finalize the contour of the abutment (Figure 8.11). The same instrument should be used to create a very defined chamfer finish line. After using this instrument there should be no sharp edges or corners remaining.

Step 2. Use the pink diamond polisher wheel to remove micro scratches from the entire abutment surface.

Step 3. Use the gray diamond polisher wheel to create a luster shine on the entire abutment surface.

Note: The red diamond instrument should be used at 50,000 rpm. No irrigation or coolant is needed. Always apply very light pressure while using this instrument. The pink and gray diamond polishers should be used at no more than 5000 rpm. *Do not* apply pressure while using these instruments. Establishing

a light contact between the polisher and abutment surface is a must. Strokes should be either away from you or toward you to maximize the luster shine result.

INTRA-ORAL ADJUSTMENT TECHNIQUES FOR A ZIRCONIA ABUTMENT

The Vitality friction grip diamond kit has been designed for adjusting ceramic materials including but not limited to sintered and non-sintered zirconia abutments in the mouth (Figure 8.12). It can also be used with a laboratory turbine for extra-oral use.

Using electroplating techniques, the Vitality instruments are made of specially sized diamond grains. This gives them friction grip capabilities as well making them application specific. The turbine handpiece, or red contra angle, should provide an rpm range of 250,000 to 300,000. Minimum contact pressure (less than 2 N) and constant irrigation is required during use (a minimum of 50 ml/min). Note that excessive pressure will generate too much heat, causing micro cracks to the abutment.

Gross Reduction Instruments

The blue diamond instruments are used for gross reduction (Figure 8.13). These blue diamonds are less aggressive than the green diamonds and are medium grained. They can be safely used for adjusting zirconia abutments. However there is a risk of chipping when adjusting aluminum oxide abutments.

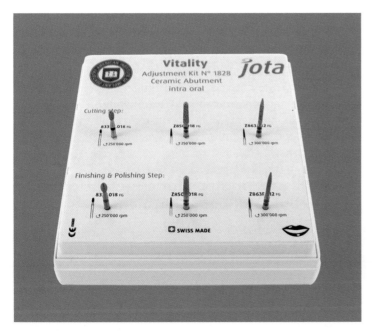
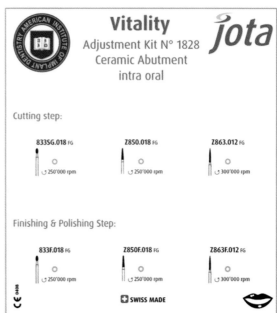

Figure 8.12 Vitality friction grip diamond kit for zirconia abutments.

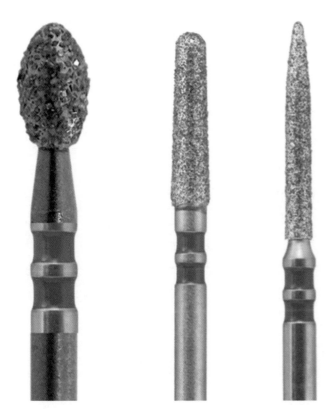

Figure 8.13 Blue band diamond instruments for the gross reduction of zirconia abutments: blue pear shaped, blue chamfer, and blue long flame shaped.

- *Blue pear shaped:* This should mainly be used to reduce zirconia abutment volume and gross reduction of incisal and lingual surfaces. This instrument should not be used for defined reduction. It is suitable for gross reduction of zirconia but can result in chipping of the abutment edge in aluminum oxide ceramic abutments.
- *Blue chamfer:* This should be used to create a chamfer finish line.
- *Blue long flame shaped:* This should be used to create the desired taper and angle between the mesial and distal surfaces.

Note: All of these blue instruments should be used at 250,000 rpm. To maximize their performance, they should be replaced after 10 uses.

Finishing Instruments

The red band diamond instruments are fine grained and using them for finishing zirconia abutment is very safe and user friendly (Figure 8.14). They will not cause edge chipping and will remove any roughness left on the surface of the abutment by the blue diamonds.

- *Red pear shaped:* This should be used for the defined reduction of incisal and lingual surfaces.
- *Red chamfer:* This should be used for the final chamfer finish line.

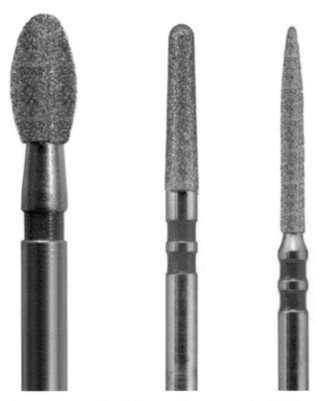

Figure 8.14 Red band diamond instruments for finishing zirconia abutments: red pear shaped, red chamfer, and red long flame shaped.

• *Red long flame shaped:* This should be used to create the final taper and angle between the mesial and distal surfaces.

Note: All of these instruments should be used at 250,000 rpm. To maximize their performance they should be replaced after 10 adjustments. Some the zirconia implant manufacturers recommend using only red diamonds for adjusting their one-piece implants.

Adjustment Steps for a Prefabricated Zirconia Implant Abutment

Gross Reduction

Step 1. Mark the labial or lingual surface of the abutment before starting gross reduction (Figure 8.15). You can use a marker or use the blue chamfer or blue long flame-shaped instrument to mark the labial and lingual surfaces.

> **Note**: If using the blue diamond for marking *do not* reduce the ceramic abutment aggressively, just mark the surface.

Step 2. Use the blue pear-shaped diamond to reduce abutment height, as well as the lingual surface (Figure 8.16). Skip this step if you are modifying an abutment with thin walls.

Step 3. The blue long flamed instrument should be used to reduce the interproximal surfaces of the

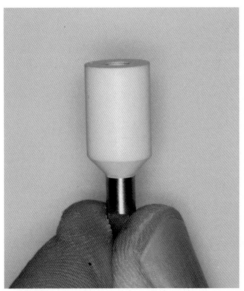
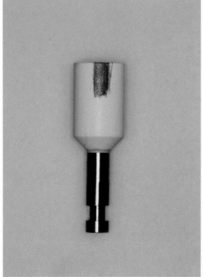
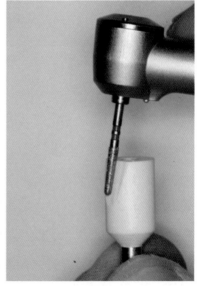

Figure 8.15 Marking the labial surface of the abutment.

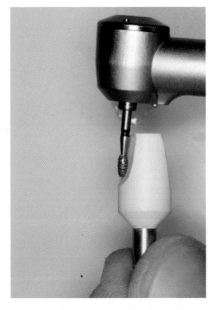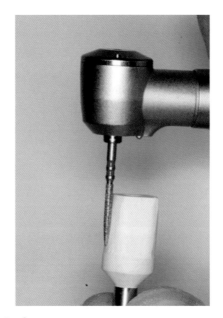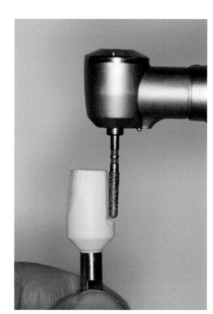

Figure 8.16 Gross reduction of a zirconia abutment.

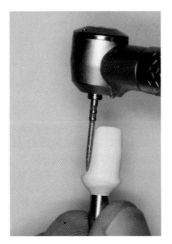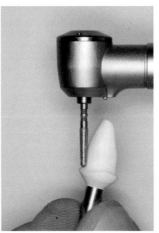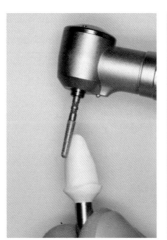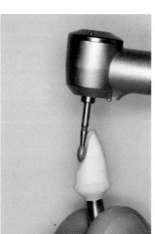

Figure 8.17 Finishing a prepared zirconia abutment.

abutment. A taper between the interproximal walls should form.

Step 4. Use the blue chamfer to establish a chamfer finish line. This instrument can be used to round up any sharp edges.

Note: These instruments should be used at 250,000 rpm with light pressure during grinding

($<2\,$N). Always use irrigation (a minimum of 50 ml/min is recommended).

Finishing

Step 1. Use the red long flame-shaped diamond instrument to finalize the interproximal taper (Figure 8.17).

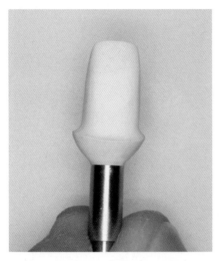 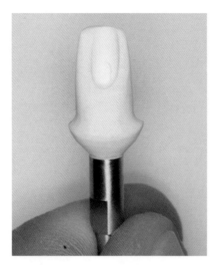 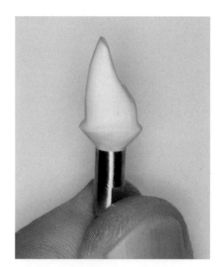

Figure 8.18 The final prepared zirconia abutment.

Step 2. The red chamfer diamond should be used to create a very defined chamfer finish line. It is also used to reduce and eliminate the scratches left by the blue diamond on the different surfaces of the abutment.

Step 3. Use the red pear diamond to define the shape and contour of the lingual surface. Since this is the last step, after using this instrument there should be no sharp edges or corners left on the ceramic abutment (Figure 8.18).

Note: These instruments should be used at 250,000 rpm with light pressure (<2 N). Use irrigation (a minimum of 50 ml/min is recommended).

REFERENCES AND FURTHER READING

Biomet-3i Restorative Manual. http://biomet3i.co.uk/Resource%20Center/Manuals%20And%20Guidelines/Restorative%20Manual_CATRM.pdf (last accessed May 2014).

Jota Vitality Manual 1828. http://www.globaldentalshop.com/product/implant-abutment-adjustment-kits/zirconia-intra-oral-kit-1828/ (last accessed May 2014).

Jota Vitality Manual 1827. http://www.globaldentalshop.com/product/implant-abutment-adjustment-kits/zirconia-intra-oral-kit-1827/ (last accessed May 2014).

Jota Vitality Manual 1826. http://www.globaldentalshop.com/product/implant-abutment-adjustment-kits/zirconia-intra-oral-kit-1826/ (last accessed May 2014).

Komet. Zir Diamonds instruction for use. http://kometprint.com/412100_GBL_D/gb/?startpage=106 (last accessed May 2014).

Komet. General instructions for use and safety recommendations for the application of rotary and oscillating dental instruments http://kometprint.com/412100_GBL_D/gb/?startpage=106 (last accessed May 2014).

Straumann prosthetic procedures. http://www.straumann.us/content/dam/internet/straumann_us/resources/guidemanual/handling-instructions/en/uslit-232-bone-level-prosthetic-procedures-manual/uslit232.pdf (last accessed May 2014).

9

Abutment Preparation Techniques for One-Piece Titanium and Zirconia Implants

Hamid R. Shafie[1] and Mary L. Ballard[2]

[1]Washington Hospital Center, Department of Oral and Maxillofacial Surgery, Washington, DC; and American Institute of Implant Dentistry, Washington, DC
[2]Private Practice, Washington, DC

INTRODUCTION

The original Branemark protocol for the placement of dental implants was based on a two-piece implant and a two-stage procedure. Although this has been a predictably successful methodology, researchers have consistently worked to establish techniques to shorten the overall treatment time and improve esthetic outcomes while maintaining successful osseointegration. With the advent of advanced surface characteristics, the time needed for predictable osseointegration has shortened. As the concept of immediate loading has gained acceptance (Atieh et al. 2010; Tortamano et al. 2010; Den Hartog et al. 2011), the one-piece implant has become a viable option. The one-piece implant incorporates the implant body, a transmucosal element, and a restorative abutment into a single structure. As the abutment is present in the oral cavity from the time of placement, some degree of immediate loading is inherent. Studies continue to emerge that demonstrate that one-piece implants have a comparable survival rate to their traditional two-piece counterparts

and that they can be a predictable restoration in implant dentistry (Borgonovo et al. 2010; Froum et al. 2011; Sohn et al. 2011).

There are many advantages thought to be gained by the one-piece design. Because the internal implant abutment connective features are eliminated (Figure 9.1), small-diameter titanium implants as narrow as 3.0 mm can be manufactured without significantly increasing the risk of fracture (Allum et al. 2008). This has allowed appropriately sized implants to be used in sites that can be otherwise too narrow for conventional implant sizes, such as the mandibular incisor and maxillary lateral incisor areas (Figure 9.2).

It should be noted that one-piece implants with less than a 3.0 mm diameter are produced – so-called "mini-implants" – but they are not categorized as permanent implants and are not recommended for the retention of crowns or dentures. They will not be the focus of discussion in this chapter.

With the elimination of the abutment screw, the one-piece titanium implant can actually be stronger than a two-piece counterpart of similar diameter

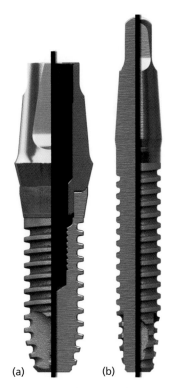

Figure 9.1 Comparison of one- and two-piece implants. (a) Two-piece design with internal components that allow thinner titanium walls. (b) One-piece design composed of a solid structure of titanium. Courtesy of BioHorizons.

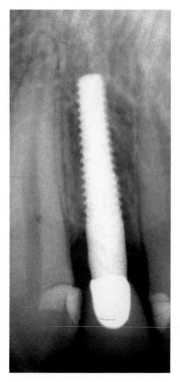

Figure 9.2 Narrow maxillary lateral incisor site restored with a 3.0 mm diameter one-piece implant. Courtesy of Dr Stephen M. Parel, DDS.

(Allum et al. 2008). Additionally, without the micro-gap inherent to two-piece implant systems, the potential for micro-leakage leading to inflammation at the implant–abutment interface is eliminated. Further, the biologic width created around one-piece implants has dimensions closer to those of natural teeth than two-piece implants, which results in a more coronally located gingival margin (Hermann et al. 2001). As one-piece implants require a single-stage procedure, there is no need for a second surgery stage where manipulation of the crestal soft tissues and bone would usually occur. A second procedure will inherently induce inflammation and has the potential to precipitate crestal bone loss. Accomplishing all the surgical steps in one procedure also reduces the overall patient discomfort associated with treatment. Moreover, the lack of total component parts needed during treatment with a one-piece implant system can lower the overall cost incurred.

One-piece implants are currently manufactured from commercially pure (CP) titanium, titanium alloy, and zirconia. There is an ever-expanding number of companies producing one-piece implants; however only a few select designs will be covered in this text.

The titanium designs discussed here have been chosen because they are part of the new generation of one-piece implants. The main distinguishing factor that separates the new generation is the inclusion of advanced surface characteristics on the implant body. These treatments, which produce increased protein binding to the implant surface, allow for immediate or early loading.

The new generation of titanium one-piece implants was introduced by Nobel Biocare with their NobelDirect® design, which utilizes their TiUnite™ surface. TiUnit is said to roughen the surface through a spark anodization process. Zimmer began producing a one-piece implant featuring their Microtexture MTX™ surface, produced by grit blasting the machined titanium implant surface with hydroxyapatite particles, followed by washing in non-etching acid and distilled water baths to remove the residual blasting material. BioHorizons also began producing a one-piece implant with a roughened surface from a blasting and acid-washing process known as the RBT (resorbable blast texturing) process.

In the new generation of titanium one-piece implants, developments have also been made in implant

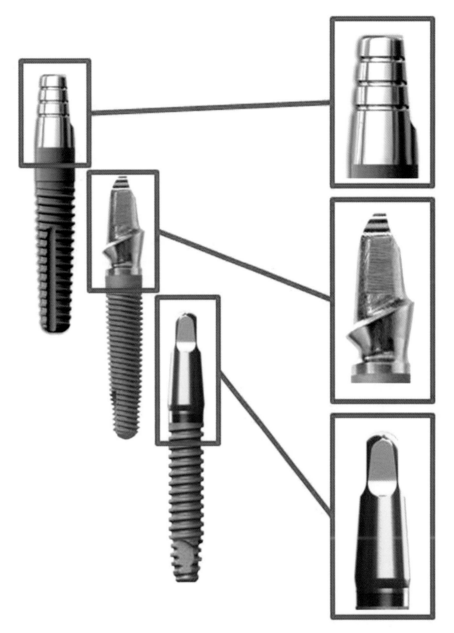

Figure 9.3   Abutment designs of selected titanium one-piece implants: Nobel BioCare NobelDirect 3.0 implant (top); Zimmer One-Piece implant (middle); BioHorizons One-Piece 3.0 implant (bottom).

macro-geometry. Companies such as Zimmer and Bio-Horizons have enhanced the design of the abutment portion of the one-piece implant (Figure 9.3).

Zimmer introduced abutments with pre-prepared chamfer margins in order to decrease chairside preparation time and decrease heat generation at the implant surface. BioHorizons modified the abutment by including a titanium nitrite coating, which is thought to increase the esthetics of the final restoration by masking the dark hue of the titanium with a more natural color.

The zirconia one-piece implant designs covered in this text have been included because they were among the first uses of zirconia as an alternative to titanium in the implant dentistry. The Z-Systems Z-Look3 Evo® implant features a sand-blasted surface; however, the current European version of the implant utilizes a SLM (surface laser modified) surface. This process of blasting and laser etching is currently pending Food and Drug Administration (FDA) approval with plans to be available on the US market in late 2012. The Bredent whiteSKY™ implant also features a sand-blasted surface, while the Oral Iceberg Cera-Root™ implants are treated with an acid-etch process known as ICE Surface™. Since the surfaces currently available on zirconia implants do not qualify as advanced surface characteristics, they may have a slower increase in secondary stability and should be subjected to a protected load protocol during healing, as described later in the chapter.

One-piece implants have been shown to successfully osseointegrate, have good long-term survival rates, and have produced excellent esthetics in multiple clinical studies (Borgonovo et al. 2010; Froum et al. 2011; Sohn et al. 2011). In order to understand the clinical success of the one-piece implant it is important to analyze their geometry at the macro- and micro-level, as well as their indications for use and the proper surgical technique required for their placement.

MATERIAL SCIENCE OF ONE-PIECE IMPLANTS

Zirconia originated in 1789 as the discovery of German chemist M. H. Klaproth. However, it was only introduced into dentistry a few decades ago: a product of the increasing desire for highly esthetic restorations. Zirconia has found many applications in dentistry, but has only recently become a prominent figure on the implant dentistry stage. Other ceramics, such as aluminum oxide, were used in the early stages of implant dentistry and were able to osseointegrate and provide esthetic restorations, but did not have the mechanical strength to withstand long-term bite forces. These early ceramics fell out of favor due to their shortcom-

ings and titanium became the mainstay for implant manufacturing.

With recent advances in the chemical processing of zirconia, it has become the first ceramic material in dental implantology able to withstand long-term loading, and subsequently has become an attractive alternative to titanium (Kohal et al. 2002, 2011; Silva et al. 2009). Zirconia has a white hue that can effectively mimic the shade of natural teeth and eliminate the unsightly gingival discoloration often encountered with titanium implants in the esthetic zone. Furthermore, zirconia has not only been shown to have similar bone–implant contact percentages as titanium (Koch et al. 2010; Stadlinger et al. 2010), but also a lesser degree of bacterial adhesion and plaque accumulation. This may have implications for the likelihood of developing peri-implantitis (Scarano et al. 2004). Zirconia has also been noted to foster excellent soft tissue attachment due to its strong biocompatibility (Stadlinger et al. 2010). Based on these properties, zirconia has demonstrated its utility as a viable alternative to titanium.

The zirconia used in dentistry today is not merely the zirconium dioxide discovered in the 18th century; commercial grade zirconia has several modifications that enhance its properties. In its pure phase, zirconium dioxide has a low shear strength and is very brittle, essentially making it useless as a dental material. The addition of small amounts of aluminum oxide and yttrium oxide increase the modulus of elasticity and help to stabilize the material. When this combination is mixed with zirconium oxide in the powder state and placed in a sintering oven, a monocline crystalline structure is produced (Figure 9.4a).

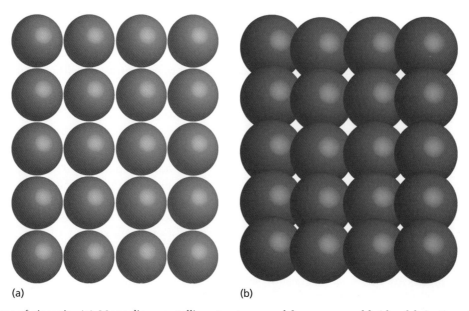

(a)   (b)

Figure 9.4 Forms of zirconia. (a) Monocline crystalline structure used for crown and bridge fabrication. (b) Tetragonal crystalline structure created after hot isostatic pressing (HIP), used for one-piece implant manufacturing.

For crown and bridge dentistry, restorations are milled from zirconia blanks and then sintered to produce this monocline structure. Although the monocline crystal is a quite strong, when cracks occur they propagate easily through the structure. As the zirconia used for implant dentistry often requires preparation with a high-speed handpiece, there is a potential to cause small cracks in the material surface. Over time, these could progress and eventually lead to material failure. This property makes monocline zirconia less desirable to use as a long-term implanted prosthesis.

In order to eliminate this issue, the zirconia used for dental implants is also exposed to a process known as HIP, or hot isostatic pressing. The high pressure under which the monocline zirconia is placed during HIP processing causes condensation of the particles and results in a tetragonal crystalline structure (Figure 9.4b). The significance of this innovation is that it imparts the ability to impede crack propagation. When the surface of HIP-processed zirconia is prepared, any micro-cracks that may result are quickly stabilized as tetragonal particles expand within the monocline structure to fill the void. This self-repairing property is also known as the "airbag effect" (Figure 9.5).

In order to manufacture zirconia dental implants, HIP-processed tetragonal zirconia blanks are milled into the desired implant shape (Figure 9.6).

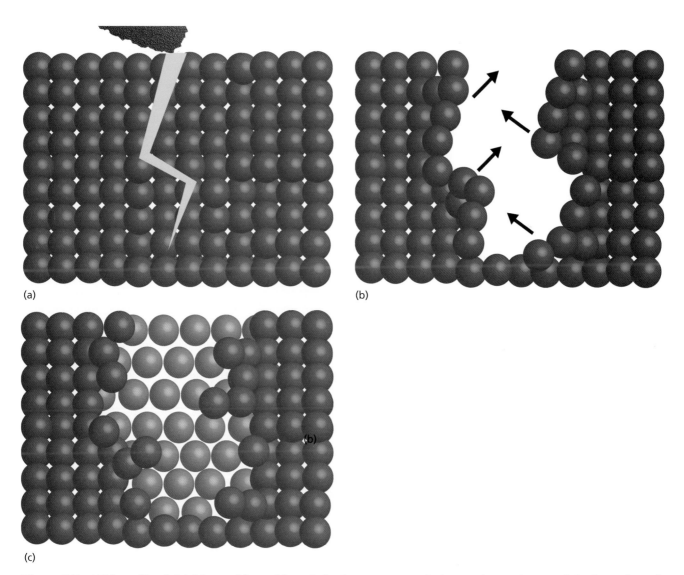

Figure 9.5 "Airbag effect." (a) Diamond bur without irrigation or proper grit size causing a micro-crack in the surface of tetragonal zirconia. (b) Micro-crack created in the surface of the tetragonal zirconia structure. Adjacent tetragonal crystals are induced to transform to monocline structure. (c) Transformation of the tetragonal crystals into a monocline structure to fill the void and halt crack propagation.

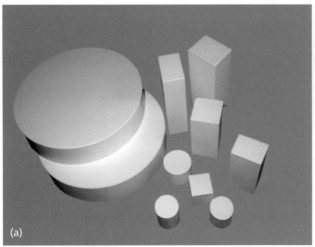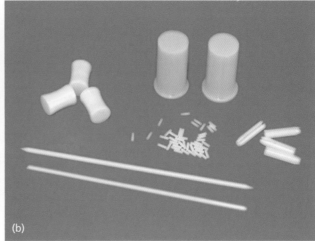

Figure 9.6 (a) Zirconia prior to sintering, which has a chalk-like consistency. (b) Sintered, HIP-processed zirconia blanks, which are extremely strong, are milled to create one-piece zirconia implants.

The additional stability gained by the HIP process has enabled zirconia to be used for multiple medical prosthetics with lifespans comparable to their metal-based counterparts (Kohal et al. 2002, 2011; Silva et al. 2009).

ONE-PIECE IMPLANT MACRO-GEOMETRY

Implant macro-geometry includes features such as the material used, shape of the implant body, length and width of the implant, and thread design, as well as the overall shape of the transmucosal element and restorative abutment. These elements are examined in detail as they pertain to the implant designs reviewed in this text to allow the clinician to gain an appreciation for the design features available (Table 9.1).

Nobel Biocare

Nobel Biocare NobelDirect implants were introduced in March 2004. The implants were originally produced with a 3.0 mm diameter with either a 13 or 15 mm length, known as NobelDirect 3.0 (Figure 9.7a).

Later, Nobel Biocare also produced one-piece implants with 3.5, 4.3, 5, and 6 mm diameters with 8 to 16 mm lengths, known as NobelDirect Groovy, Oval, and Posterior. Although still available, these designs will not be the focus of this chapter.

The NobelDirect 3.0 implants are produced from cold-worked grade 4 CP titanium. The implant body

has a tapered design with a 2.0 mm diameter at the apex and is treated with Nobel Biocare's TiUnite surface. The implant features a buttress micro-thread with a 0.6 mm thread pitch. The NobelDirect 3.0 implant has a straight transmucosal element which is 3 mm in height, measured from the most coronal aspect of the threaded portion to just above the apical extent of the machined surface. This area, up to the beginning of the polished portion, is also treated with the TiUnite surface. The rationale for roughening the surface of the transmucosal portion was to create a stronger soft tissue seal, based on literature that suggests a shorter contact epithelium is created at oxidized, acid-etched surfaces (Glauser et al. 2005). The abutment portion of the implant is 5 mm in height and has a tapered cylindrical shape with one flattened portion to act as an antirotational element. The abutment is manufactured with a smooth, machined surface and does not have a predetermined restorative finish line.

Zimmer

The Zimmer One-Piece implant, introduced in 2007, is produced from grade 5 titanium alloy (Figure 9.7b). The implants are produced in 3.0, 3.7, and 4.7 mm diameters with lengths ranging from 10 to 16 mm. The implant body has a tapered design, with shorter implants having larger degrees of taper. The 3.0 mm diameter implants have a triple-lead V-shaped thread design, whereas the 3.7 and 4.7 mm diameter implants are given a double-lead V-shaped thread. The entire implant body is treated with the MTX surface, which includes the threaded portion plus an unthreaded area

Table 9.1 Comparison of the design elements of selected one-piece implants

	Company	Material	Body shape	Sizes	Thread design	Transmucosal design	Abutment shape
Titanium implants	Nobel Biocare NobelDirect®	Grade 4 commercially pure titanium	Tapered	3.0 mm width with 13 or 15 mm length 3.5, 4.3, 5, or 6 mm widths with 8, 10, 13, or 16 mm lengths	Buttress micro-thread	Straight	Tapered cylinder
	Zimmer One-Piece	Grade 5 titanium alloy	Tapered	3.0, 3.7, or 4.7 mm widths with 10, 11.5, 13, or 16 mm lengths	3.0 mm diameter, V-shaped triple lead 3.7/4.7 mm diameter, V-shaped double lead	Flared	Tapered cylinder with angled finish line, straight, and 17-degree angled versions
	BioHorizons One-Piece 3.0	Grade 5 titanium alloy	Parallel walled	3.0 mm width with 12, 15, or 18 mm length	Single-helix, modified square shaped	Straight	Tapered cylinder coated with titanium nitrite
Zirconia implants	Z-Systems Z-Look3 Evo®	Zirconium oxide TZP-A BIO-HIP	Parallel walled	3.6 mm width with 10 or 11.5 mm length 4 mm width with 8, 10, 11.5, or 13 mm length 5/5.4 mm width with 10 or 11.5 mm length 5/6 mm width with 8, 10, 11.5, or 13 mm length	Single helix, V-shaped	Tulip shaped	Tapered cylinder with flat finish line
	Bredent whiteSKY™	Brezirkon	Conical–cylindrical hybrid	3.5 mm width with 10, 12, 14, or 16 mm length 4 mm width with 8, 10, 12, 14, or 16 mm length 4.5 mm width with 8, 10, 12 or 14 mm length	Double-helix	Straight	Tapered cylinder with flat finish line
	Oral Iceberg CeraRoot™	Yttrium-reinforced zirconium dioxide	Varies based on design	Five designs indicated to replace specific teeth with 10, 12, or 14 mm lengths	Single-helix, rounded V-shape	Varies	Anatomically shaped with scalloped finish line

at the coronal aspect. A 0.5 mm machined collar forms the base of the transmucosal element. The transmucosal area of the implant has a flared design and is 1.2 mm in height at the buccal margin. The flared design is thought to allow greater tissue thickness circumferentially at the alveolar crest to mask the implant's gray hue and to produce a more natural emergence profile. The implants are produced with either straight or 17-degree angled abutments, which are 4–6 mm in height for the 3.0 mm diameter implants (Figure 9.8).

The abutments are manufactured with a pre-established chamfer finish line. The finish line is angled along the circumference of the abutment, with the more apical aspect corresponding with the facial crown margin. The purpose of including the pre-established finish line was to decrease the need for chairside preparation, which is thought to produce heat and damage the adjacent bone, potentially compromising osseointegration. For the 3.0 mm diameter implants, the restorative platform has 3.5 mm diameter.

BioHorizons

BioHorizons introduced the BioHorizons One-Piece 3.0 implant (formerly Maximus) in December 2003 (see Figure 9.7c). The implants are produced from grade 5 titanium alloy and are only produced in a 3.0 mm diameter with 12, 15, or 18 mm lengths. The majority of the implant body is parallel-walled with a tapered apical portion. The implants feature a modified square-shaped thread design (Figure 9.9).

The implant body is treated with their RBT surface. The implant has a predominantly straight transmucosal element with a very subtle flare at the transition to the titanium nitrite-treated surface. There is a

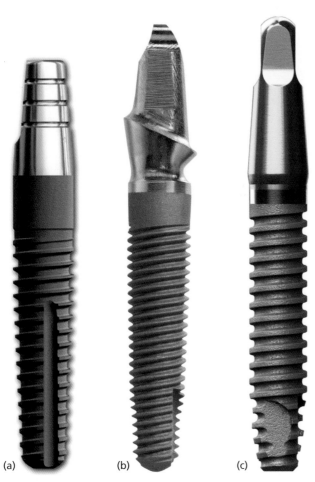

Figure 9.7 Selected titanium one-piece implant designs. (a) Nobel BioCare NobelDirect 3.0 implant. (b) Zimmer One-Piece implant. (c) BioHorizons One-Piece 3.0 implant.

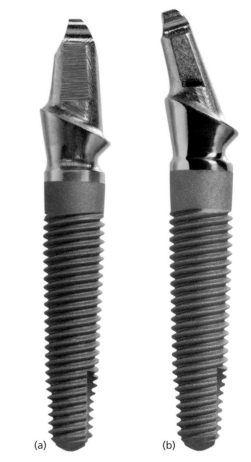

Figure 9.8 Zimmer One-Piece implants. (a) With a straight abutment. (b) With a 17-degree angled abutment.

0.7 mm machined collar just coronal to the first thread. The abutment has a tapered cylindrical shape without a restorative finish line. The abutment portion is 8 mm in height and coated with a 3-micron thick titanium nitrite coating, giving it a gold hue. This surface coloration is intended to mask the titanium with a more natural color to improve the appearance of the final restoration and decrease gingival discoloration, particularly in those with a thin gingival biotype. The coronal aspect of the abutment has a narrowed portion with four flattened surfaces, which allows a stable connection between the implant and driver during placement.

Z-Systems

Implants from Z-Systems have been available in Europe since 2004 and the Z-Look3 implant, their original design, was approved for use on the American market in 2007. Z-Systems' second generation implant, the Z-Look3 Evo (Figure 9.10a), became available in

the USA in September 2011 and included changes to the implant sizes offered and the design of the abutment portion.

The original design included an insertion hex above the abutment portion which had to be ground off following placement. This element was eliminated in the second generation design to minimize the amount of preparation required for the newly placed implants. Instead, a retention groove along the side of the abutment was added. Z-Systems implants are produced from zirconia TZP-A BIO-HIP®, which is a HIP-processed zirconia. The Z-Look3 Evo implants are available in various sizes: 3.6 mm diameter with 10 and 11.5 mm lengths, 4 mm diameter with 8, 10, 11.5, and 13 mm lengths, 5 mm diameter with 5.4 mm restorative platform in either 10 or 11.5 mm lengths, or 5 mm diameter with 6 mm restorative platform in 8, 10, 11.5, and 13 mm lengths. The implant body has a parallel-walled design with an apical taper and a single-helix V-shaped thread design. The surface of the implant body is treated with a sand-blasting process, and the total length of the sand-blasted portion of the

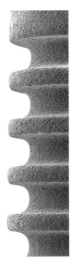

Figure 9.9 Modified square-shaped thread design of the BioHorizons One-Piece 3.0 implant.

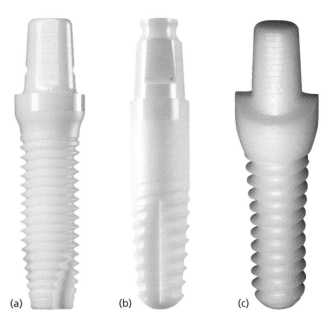

(a)   (b)   (c)

Figure 9.10 Selected zirconia one-piece implant designs. (a) Z-Systems Z-Look3 Evo implant. (b) Bredent whiteSKY implant. (c) Oral Iceberg CeraRoot implant (CeraRoot 21 design).

implant corresponds to the advertised implant length. As previously mentioned, a new surface treatment known as SLM is currently pending FDA approval and will be incorporated into the design when approved. The transmucosal area has a "tulip shape," which is essentially a convex, rounded flare that leads up to the restorative shoulder. The implant restorative abutment area has a tapered cylindrical shape with a flattened area that acts as an antirotational element during insertion. The implant shoulder is symmetric with a flat restorative finish line.

Bredent

The Bredent whiteSKY implant (Figure 9.10b) was brought to the European market in April 2006, but is not currently available in the USA. It is manufactured from Brezirkon®, Bredent's yttrium oxide-stabilized, tetragonal polycrystalline zirconium oxide. Implants are produced with 3.5, 4, and 4.5 mm diameters with lengths ranging from 8 to 16 mm. The implant body has a conical–cylindrical hybrid form, meaning that the threaded apical portion of the implant body is tapered, while the non-threaded coronal 3 mm has a cylindrical shape. The threaded portion of the implant body has a double-helix thread design, and both the unthreaded and threaded portions of the implant body have a sand-blasted surface. The implant length is measured from the apex of the implant to the coronal edge of the sand-blasted surface. The transmucosal aspect of the implant is 2 mm in height and has a straight design with a smooth, machined surface. The abutment portion of the implant is 6.8 mm in height and has a tapered cylindrical shape with a flattened side that acts as an antirotational element. There is a circumferential

groove at the most coronal aspect of the abutment, which serves to stabilize the implant within its packaging. The restorative finish line has a flat design with a restorative platform that corresponds to the implant body width for the 4.0 and 4.5 mm diameter implants. For the 3.5 mm diameter implant, the transmucosal component of the implant is slightly wider than the implant body, allowing for a 4.0 mm restorative platform at the finish line.

Oral Iceberg

Oral Iceberg is the manufacturer of CeraRoot implants (see Figure 9.10c), a unique line of yttrium-reinforced zirconium dioxide implants that were brought to the European market in 2007. They received FDA approval in January 2011 and are now being marketed in the USA. The CeraRoot system features five different implant designs (Figure 9.11), each meant to be particularly well suited for the replacement of specific teeth within the arch.

The CeraRoot 12 design is a 4.1 mm diameter implant with a threaded, parallel-walled implant body meant for use in mandibular incisor and maxillary lateral incisor sites. The CeraRoot 11 and 21 implants are similar in design; both have implant bodies with parallel-walled apical portions and flared, conical coronal portions. CeraRoot 21 implants are intended to replace maxillary central incisors as well as maxillary and mandibular canines; they feature a 4.1 mm

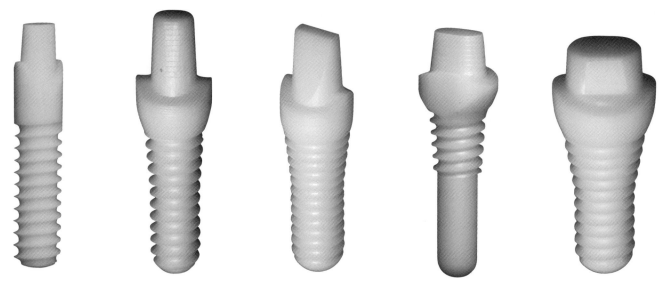

Figure 9.11   CeraRoot designs (left to right): CeraRoot 12, CeraRoot 21, CeraRoot 11, CeraRoot 14, and CeraRoot 16.

implant body diameter at the apex and a 6 mm diameter restorative platform. CeraRoot 11 implants, on the other hand, are only meant to replace maxillary central incisors and canines, and have a 4.8 mm diameter at the apex and a 6.5 mm restorative platform. CeraRoot 16 implants have a shape similar to the 11 and 21 designs with a cylindrical implant body at the apex but flared design in the coronal aspect; however, they have a wider diameter to accommodate molar sites. The implant body has a 4.8 mm diameter at the apex with an 8 mm diameter restorative platform.

The CeraRoot 14 design is quite different from the other designs. The implant has an oval cross-section at the level of the restorative platform, meant to replicate the normal cross-section of a premolar tooth. This more anatomic shape is meant to provide the best emergence profile and overall esthetic result for the replacement of premolars. Due to the non-traditional shape of this implant, it is placed with a press-fit technique, as described later in the text. For this reason, the apical portion of the implant body is not threaded, and threading on the coronal portion of the implant body is only present to further stabilize the implant during initial placement and healing.

All CeraRoot designs are available in 10, 12, or 14 mm implant body lengths. The thread design for the CeraRoot implants is a single-helix, rounded V shape, and the implant surface is treated with an acid-etching process known as ICE Surface. The transmucosal element of the implant, which is defined as the area between the most coronal thread and the most apical portion of the finish line, ranges in height from 2.5 to 3.5 mm depending on the implant design. For CeraRoot 12 implants, the transmucosal portion

is straight, while for CeraRoot 11, 21, and 16 is takes on a flared shape. In CeraRoot 14 implants, the transmucosal design may be described as more of a tulip shape. The abutment portions of the CeraRoot implants were designed to mimic the shape of a traditional crown preparation. Thus, the implants meant for incisor sites have incisor crown preparation-shaped abutments, while the molar implants have molar crown preparation-shaped abutments. Each has at least one flattened surface that acts as an anti-rotational element. The restorative finish lines are also meant to correspond to the ideal shape of traditional crown preparations. The restorative finish lines are scalloped, with the most apical portions designed to be positioned on the buccal and lingual aspects of the surgical site, while the most coronal portions of the finish line are to be placed in the mesial and distal positions.

ONE-PIECE IMPLANT MICRO-GEOMETRY

Micro-geometry in implant dentistry refers largely to the surface texture of the implant body. Having a roughened implant surface is known to enhance migration and proliferation of osteoblasts and to precipitate osseointegration (Nasatzky et al. 2003; Osathanon et al. 2011). Ideal surface roughness is thought to be in the range of 1–100 microns for the best osteoblast attachment, which ultimately results in the highest bone–implant connection. Blasting processes, which are used by multiple companies, serve to

Table 9.2 Comparison of the micro-geometry of selected one-piece implants

Company	Brand name	Process	Roughness
Nobel Biocare NobelDirect®	TiUnite™	Spark anodization	1.3 microns
Zimmer One-Piece	Microtexture (MTX)™	Blasted, acid washed	1–2 microns
BioHorizons One-Piece 3.0	Resorbable blast texturing (RBT)	Blasted with tricalcium phosphate, washed with nitric acid	60 Ra
Z-Systems Z-Look3 Evo®	None	Blasted with aluminum oxide	1.5 microns
	Surface laser modified (SLM) (pending FDA approval)	Blasted with aluminum oxide, laser modified	5.2 microns
Bredent whiteSKY™	None	Blasted	1 micron
Oral Iceberg CeraRoot™	ICE Surface™	Acid etched	1.16 microns

increase the surface area of the implant body through a subtractive process, resulting in peaks and valleys across the implant surface. Often the implant surfaces are also treated with an acid. Varying terminology exists for these processes, such as acid washing and acid etching. It should be noted that washing with an acid also results in etching the surface, so the terminology is essentially equivocal. Treatment with an acid will remove residual debris from a previously blasted implant surface in addition to etching the surface.

These processes result in a decreased contact angle, which allows better fluid flow and protein binding along the implant surface. These processes all serve to increase bone–implant contact percentages and overall stability of the implants, which ultimately results in better long-term survival. The prominent features of the micro-geometry of the designs covered in this chapter are presented in Table 9.2.

The TiUnite surface applied to Nobel Biocare Nobel-Direct implants is an electrochemical oxidation procedure which Nobel Biocare began applying to their implants in 2000. It results in a surface with a porous texture and a roughness of approximately 1.2 microns (Figure 9.12a) (Schuepbach and Glauser 2012).

The BioHorizons One-Piece 3.0 implants are treated with their RBT process, which involves blasting the implant surface with tricalcium phosphate, followed by acid washing. This results in a surface roughness of approximately 2 microns (Figure 9.12b). Zimmer One-Piece implants have surfaces treated with their

MTX process, in which the implant surface is blasted with hydroxyapatite particles, then washed in non-etching acid and distilled water baths to remove the residual blasting material. The MTX process results in a surface roughness of approximately 1–2 microns (Figure 9.12c).

As zirconia dental implants are newer to the market, the technology available for surface treatments is somewhat less sophisticated as compared with titanium at this time. Both Z-Systems Z-Look3 Evo and Bredent whiteSKY implants utilize a sand-blasting process to treat the zirconia surface (Figure 9.13a, b).

These processes result in a surface roughness of approximately 1.5 and 1 micron, respectively. The Oral Iceberg CeraRoot implants, on the other hand, are now utilizing an acid-etching process to treat the implant surface known as the ICE Surface (Figure 9.13c). The Z-Systems implants recently introduced a new FDA-approved surface characteristic known as SLM. This process consists of blasting the implant surface, then further modifying the roughness through the use of a laser (Figure 9.13d).

CASE SELECTION CRITERIA

General Considerations

Basic Principles of Implant Placement

- Adequate bone volume and density
- No evidence of pathology
- Adequate periodontal health of adjacent teeth
- Reasonable tissue health at the surgical site
- Completion of skeletal growth
- Conical root form of the extracted tooth*
- Site free of peri-apical disease or frank infection*
- Intact bony walls*
- >1mm thickness of buccal plate*

*For immediate implant placement.

Patient compliance is especially important for success in one-piece implants. The patient must be able to avoid chewing with the provisional crown or religiously wear their removable protective appliance during healing so that unfavorable forces on the implant can be limited.

Anatomic Considerations

Three-Dimensional Space Limitation

One-piece implants have been designed that can be used to replace any tooth. However, their most unique application is for narrow spaces in which traditional

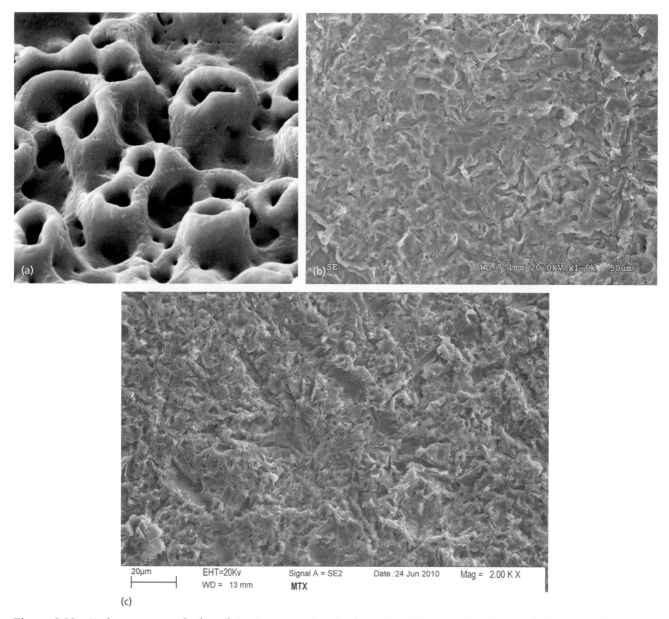

Figure 9.12 Surface textures of selected titanium one-piece implants. (a) TiUnite surface from Nobel Biocare. (b) RBT surface from BioHorizons. (c) MTX surface from Zimmer.

implant sizes would surpass the limits of the bone volume (Figures 9.14 and 9.15).

Often the buccolingual and mesiodistal dimensions of the alveolus are reduced in the maxillary and mandibular incisor areas, and placement of a standard-sized 3.5 or 4 mm diameter implant can lead to the exposure of implant threads and bone loss or damage to adjacent teeth (Sohn et al. 2011). Due to the one-piece design and greater internal bulk of material, titanium one-piece permanent implants can be manufactured with very small diameters while still maintaining excellent strength. Two-piece implants

are also currently being manufactured with 3.0 mm diameters, but will inherently have a greater risk of fracture due to their design.

The narrow-diameter implants are indicated for mandibular incisor and maxillary lateral incisor sites. They are not recommended for use in posterior sites with small mesiodistal lengths where traditional implants sizes cannot be used, or generally for the replacement of premolar or molar teeth. By using these narrow-diameter implants for the replacement of incisors, teeth with small cervical diameters can be replaced with implants of a similar diameter, which

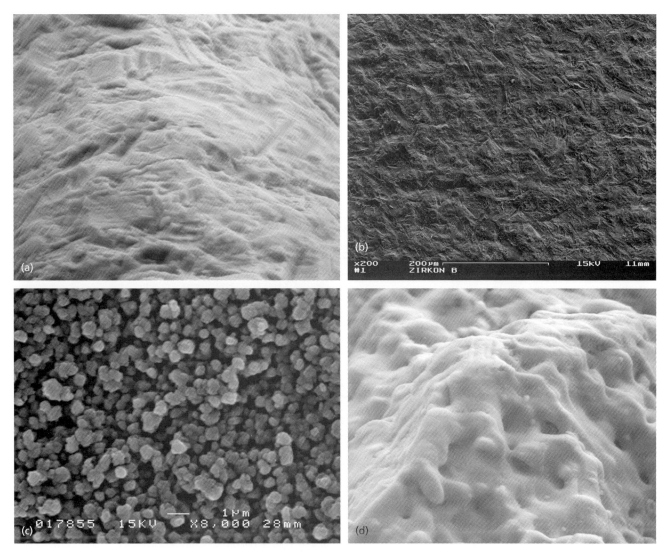

Figure 9.13 Surface textures of selected zirconia one-piece implants. (a) Z-Systems blasted surface. (b) Z-Systems SLM surface. (c) Bredent blasted surface. (d) Oral Iceberg ICE Surface.

helps to achieve the best emergence profile and esthetic result. Implants to be used within these narrow-diameter sites should be chosen to maximize the available bone height. The advent of these implants has allowed for successful implant restorations to be placed in sites previously thought to be not amenable for implant restoration or which required extensive grafting procedures or orthodontics prior to placement.

Abutment Angulation

When selecting cases for one-piece implant placement, one must consider the angulation required for the abutment and future restoration.

All of the one-piece implant designs discussed in this chapter have an abutment that is orientated along the long axis of the implant body, with the exception of the Zimmer One-Piece, which has either a straight or a 17-degree angled abutment. The anatomic shape of the available bone will dictate the position of the implant body. In a clinical scenario where it appears that an abutment angulation in excess of 15–20 degrees will be required, one-piece implants are not appropriate (Figure 9.16). Although abutments can be customized to a certain degree (as discussed later in this chapter), surpassing these limits compromises the retention of the restoration and the structural integrity of the implant.

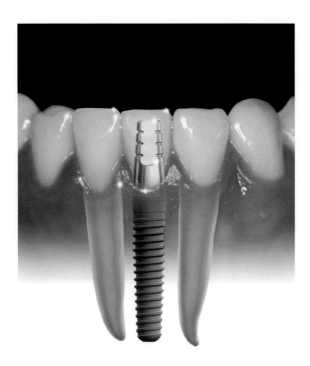

Figure 9.14   Narrow-diameter one-piece implant replacing a mandibular incisor. Courtesy of Nobel Biocare.

Biomechanical Considerations

Preferred Occlusal Scheme

Regardless of the type of one-piece implant chosen or the method of provisionalization, the patient must have adequate occlusion to allow for the implant to heal in the least traumatic environment and for the final restoration to not be subjected to unfavorable forces. One-piece implants are contraindicated in patients with severely collapsed bites, deep bites, or anterior cross-bite, or in patients with a steep incisal guidance (Figure 9.17).

One-piece implants are also not recommended in patients with severe parafunctional habits including bruxism that might cause excessive loading and adversely affect osseointegration.

Primary Stability

The exposed abutment portion of the implant will be subjected to some amount of loading from the time of placement, so a high primary stability is important. Since an implant stability quotient (ISQ) cannot be obtained for one-piece implants, a calibrated torque wrench should always be used during placement and at least 35 N-cm should be attained. Attempting to maintain an implant with a low primary stability during healing under these condi-

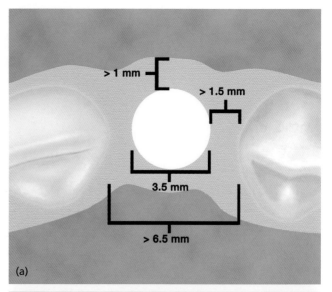

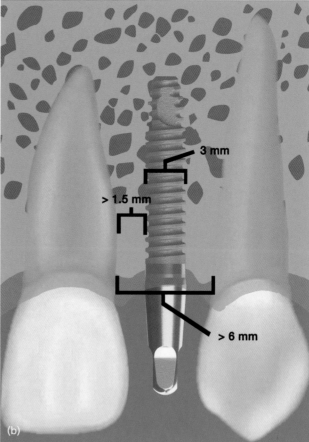

Figure 9.15   Space requirements for one-piece implants. (a) A minimum of 1–2 mm of buccal and lingual bone is necessary, with 1.5–2 mm of bone between the implant and adjacent teeth. (b) A minimum of 1.5–2 mm of bone is necessary between the implant and adjacent teeth.

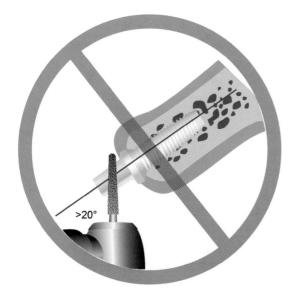

Figure 9.16 Severe angulation of a one-piece implant which would require excessive removal of the abutment structure to allow for restoration. Although the implant is correctly positioned in bone, the bony anatomy has led to excessive angulation of the abutment portion of the implant.

tions is inherently risky and may lead to higher rates of implant failure. When primary stability cannot be achieved, company literature suggests that either a graft should be placed for a future attempt at one-piece implant placement, or a two-piece submerged implant should be used.

Design of the Final Prosthesis

When the case requires the replacement of multiple teeth with small-diameter one-piece implants (3.0 or 3.6 mm), it is preferable to replace each tooth with an implant. Caution should be taken when constructing fixed partial denture designs on narrow implants. Cantilevered restorations are contraindicated under all circumstances, regardless of implant diameter. In cases where multiple adjacent small-diameter implants are to be used, planning for a splinted final restoration is preferable.

One-Piece Titanium Versus Zirconia Implants

Table 9.3 summarizes indications for the use of titanium as opposed to zirconia for one-piece implants.

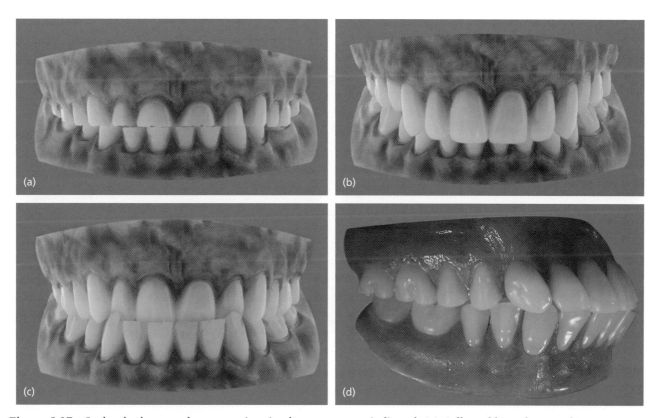

Figure 9.17 Occlusal schemes where one-piece implants are contraindicated. (a) Collapsed bite. (b) Deep bite. (c) Anterior cross-bite. (d) Steep incisal guidance.

Table 9.3 Generalized indications for the use of titanium and zirconia in one-piece implants

	Titanium	Zirconia
Scalloped, thin gingival biotype	Not recommended	✓
Thick and flat gingival biotype	✓	✓
Space limitation that requires 3 mm diameter implant	✓	✗
Immediate load option	✓	Not recommended
Patient with metal allergy	✗	✓

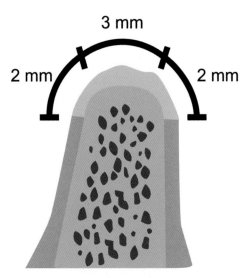

Figure 9.18 Minimum amount of attached gingiva needed for the placement of a 3 mm diameter implant with a flapless technique. The gingiva over the implant site would be lost, leaving 2 mm of attached tissue remaining on either side of the alveolus.

SURGICAL TECHNIQUES

General Considerations

Flapped Versus Flapless Techniques

After the decision has been made to use a one-piece implant, the surgical approach must be determined. Both flapped and flapless techniques for the placement of one-piece implants have been shown to be successful (Froum et al. 2011). None of the manufacturers of the implants presented in this text have indicated within their literature that flapless surgery is contraindicated for their products. Prior to using a flapless technique, the preoperative bone volume and amount of gingiva should be taken into consideration. With a flapless technique, the gingiva overlying the site will be lost during the procedure. In cases where the attached gingiva is limited, the tissue lost by using a flapless technique may be unacceptable. The amount of tissue expected to be lost from using a flapless technique should correspond to the width of the implant. At least 2 mm of attached gingiva should be present both buccally and lingually after tissue healing when measured from the marginal gingiva to the mucogingival junction. Bearing in mind these figures, for a 3 mm diameter implant, the surgical site should have at least 7 mm of attached gingiva buccolingually along the alveolus to be appropriate for a flapless technique (Figure 9.18).

Furthermore, if bone volume is very limited, it may be especially challenging to use a flapless technique. As with two-piece dental implants, at least 1.5–2 mm of bone should be present between the implant and adjacent teeth, and at least 1–2 mm of buccal and lingual bone should be preserved. For a 3 mm diameter implant, the mesiodistal distance necessary for placement is 6 mm, and the buccolingual

width necessary is 5 mm. When the preoperative clinical and radiographic measurements approach these distances, the precision required for appropriate placement may be especially challenging with a flapless technique. Preoperative three-dimensional imaging is generally recommended for flapless surgery to verify the bone volume prior to implant placement.

Immediate Placement

The placement of dental implants into fresh extraction sockets in the esthetic zone has been shown to be a successful methodology by many authors (Crespi et al. 2008; Mijiritsky et al. 2009). For immediate placement of an implant following tooth extraction to be predictably successful, the extraction socket needs to have four intact bony walls and a buccal plate thickness of at least 1 mm. To decrease the chance of damage to the existing bony walls during extraction, an atraumatic extraction technique should be utilized. A manual periotome or piezoelectric unit with a periotome tip may facilitate this process (Figure 9.19).

Any granulation tissue from the extraction site should be thoroughly debrided. In sites where there is evidence of an active or chronic infectious process, implant placement should be deferred. The bony walls should then be meticulously checked with a perio probe for fracture or fenestrations.

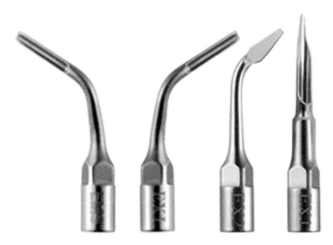

Figure 9.19 Periotome tips for a piezosurgery unit. Courtesy of EMS.

Nobel Biocare NobelDirect 3.0 Surgical Protocol

For NobelDirect 3.0 implants, the surgical procedure begins by preparing the initial osteotomy with the use of a 1.5-mm diameter pilot drill directly through the gingiva (Figure 9.20) (Nobel Biocare 2005; Parel and Schow 2005). A drill guide is available that mimics the shape of the implant abutment and is placed over the pilot drill to aid in optimal positioning.

When used to depth with the drill guide in place, an osteotomy of 8–10 mm depth will be created, depending on tissue thickness. In cases where narrow-diameter implants are to be used, the positioning of the initial pilot osteotomy is of critical importance as there is a limited amount of bone in these areas and a limited number of steps during which adjustments can be made prior to implant placement. In the optimal buccolingual position, the center of the implant abutment is at the same trajectory as the former incisal edge.

After the initial osteotomy has been made, either a flap is reflected or a tissue punch used to remove tissue from the site. A tissue punch guide is available for this purpose. Nobel Biocare indicates that flapped surgery should be used in cases where adequate bone volume has not been confirmed, when direct vision of anatomic landmarks is necessary, or when a facial connective tissue graft is to be used.

A 2 mm diameter drill known as the "soft bone" drill is then used to the planned implant depth. In cases where soft bone is present, the site is then ready for implant placement. In sites where dense bone is present, the use of the slightly wider "dense bone" drill is the final step. This drill is a "stepped" drill, with a

2 mm diameter at the tip, a 2.25 mm wide mid-section, and a 3 mm diameter near the shank.

The implant driver fits snugly over the abutment portion of the implant and the flattened side of the abutment allows the implant to be rotated. The implant can then be driven either by the handpiece or using a manual torque wrench. The torque value should be between 35 and 45 N-cm. The implant should be placed such that the flattened side of the abutment portion faces buccally.

The implant depth is not specifically addressed in the surgical guide, but generally speaking the implant should be placed such that the threaded portion is entirely within the bone but not so deep that the height of the abutment portion is too short for adequate crown retention. Generally there will be at least 1–2 mm of the TiUnite-treated surface visible above the crestal bone when the implant is positioned. The surgical protocol is illustrated in Figure 9.20, and a clinical case demonstrating the placement and restoration of a Nobel Biocare NobelDirect implant is demonstrated in Figure 9.21.

Zimmer One-Piece Surgical Protocol

The Zimmer One-Piece has a similar surgical protocol (Figure 9.22) (Zimmer Dental 2007).

Zimmer recommends a conventional flapped technique for the procedure, although the use of a flapless protocol is supported when adequate bone volume has been established. The initial drill is 2.1/1.6 mm in diameter and is used to a depth of 7 mm at the intended implant site. Once the initial osteotomy has been made, a try-in implant that replicates the abutment can be placed in the site. Based on its position, multiple decisions should be made. The necessary size of the future implant can be made, and the decision of whether to use a straight or angled version of the implant can be made. In addition, if the geometry is such that the angulation required would be greater than that a one-piece implant can accommodate, a two-piece implant protocol may be employed. Once the decision has been made to proceed with a one-piece implant of a particular size, the procedure can be resumed.

The osteotomy is then extended to the planned depth with the 2.3 mm diameter drill, and then further enlarged with the 2.8/2.4 mm diameter drill. For type III–IV bone, a 3.0 mm implant may then be placed. In the case of dense, type I–II bone in the site, a bone tap should be used at 15–30 rpm prior to implant placement. If a larger diameter implant is required, additional steps must be followed prior to placement. The implants can be placed with either a handpiece or ratchet, and the seating torque should

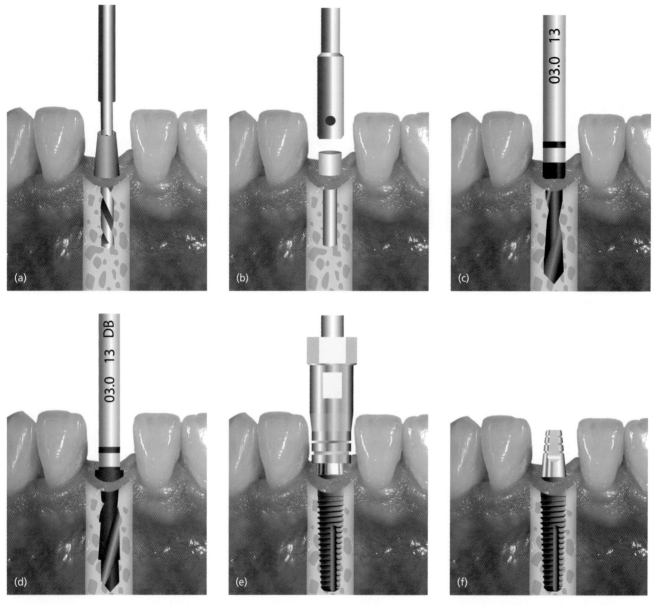

Figure 9.20 Nobel Biocare NobelDirect 3.0 surgical protocol. (a) Initial osteotomy being established with a pilot drill. The drill guide mimics the shape of the implant abutment. (b) Tissue punch guide placed into the osteotomy, with the tissue punch ready to be used. (c) Soft bone drill. (d) Dense bone drill (optional). (e) NobelDirect 3.0 implant being inserted with the implant driver. (f) NobelDirect 3.0 implant in place.

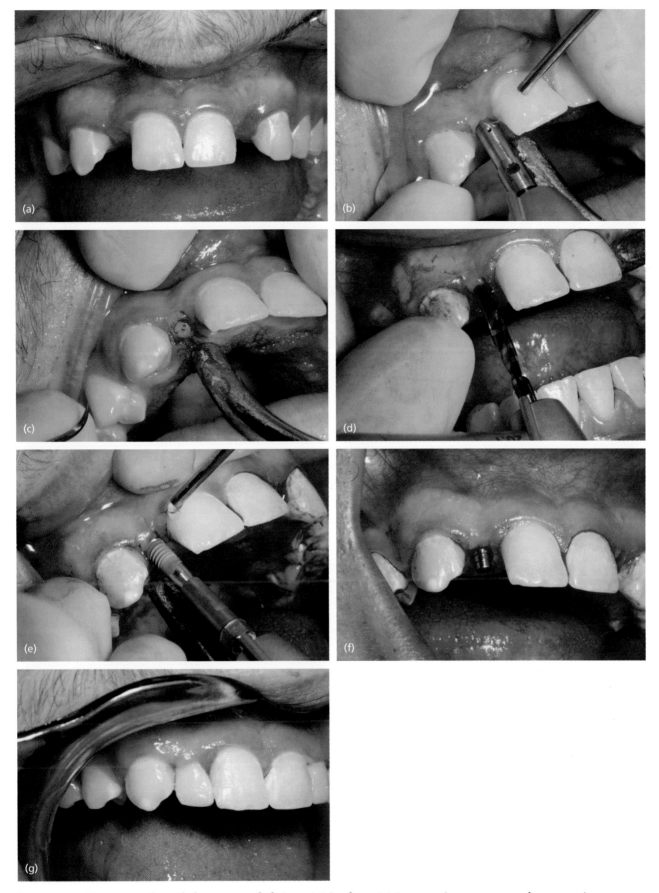

Figure 9.21 Placement of a Nobel Biocare NobelDirect 3.0 implant. (a) Preoperative appearance demonstrating a very limited space in the maxillary lateral incisor sites. (b) Use of the tissue punch for a flapless technique. (c) Tissue to be removed for a flapless technique. (d) Creation of an osteotomy. (e) Implant being inserted. (f) Implant appearance at the initial placement. (g) Provisional crown in place at 1 week post-op.

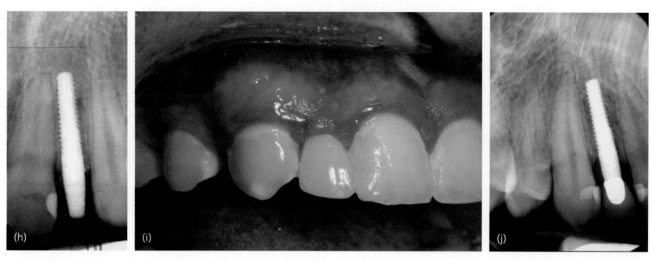

Figure 9.21 (*Continued*) (h) Radiograph at 1 week post-op. (i) Final restoration in place. (j) Radiograph after delivery of the final restoration. Courtesy of Dr Stephen M. Parel, DDS.

be no greater than 35 N-cm according to company literature.

The implant driver covers the abutment portion of the implant when engaged, so a marking line on the driver is present to aid in proper positioning of the mid-buccal margin area of the implant. The more apical contour of the angled prosthetic finish line should be placed towards the buccal side of the site. Following the company's recommendations, the implants should be placed with the entire MTX-treated surface within the bone.

BioHorizons One-Piece 3.0 Surgical Protocol

For the placement of BioHorizons One-Piece 3.0 implants, the company states that either a flapless or flapped procedure can be appropriate based on the clinician's judgment (BioHorizons 2010). The sequencing of steps involved in implant placement are demonstrated in Figure 9.23 and clinically in Figure 9.24.

The procedure is started with the use of an alignment drill, which is a sharp, narrow drill of 5 mm length. Similar to those from other companies, this drill is used to determine the ideal location of the implant. This drill is slightly different, however, in that it also prepares the crestal bone surface to provide a flattened stop for the remaining drills in the sequence. After the small initial osteotomy is made, a corresponding trial implant can be placed in the site that mimics the restorative abutment and allows for evaluation of the future implant position. The alignment drill can also be used to revise the initial position with its side-cutting action when necessary. The osteotomy is then deepened to the expected

implant length with a 2.0 mm diameter drill. This drill is pre-measured to correspond with the length of the implant, and is equipped with a stop to ensure proper depth.

For soft type II–IV bone, BioHorizons recommends that implants are placed after this step. When more dense (type I) bone is encountered, it is recommended to also use the 2.5 mm diameter drill to depth prior to placement. In cases where primarily cortical bone is noted, a bone tap at less than 30 rpm may also be used. Depending on operator preference, the implant may be then placed with either a hand ratchet or handpiece to a final insertion torque of 35–50 N-cm. The proper depth of the implant is within a 1.5 mm zone delineated by the top of the surface treatment at the flare of the abutment portion (Figure 9.25).

Z-Systems Z-Look3 Evo Surgical Protocol

Z-Systems currently offers Z-Look3 implants, as well as a newer line known as Z-Look3 Evo (Z-Systems 2008). For the purposes of this text, the Z-Look3 Evo surgical protocol will be reviewed. The steps involved are demonstrated in Figure 9.26 and a clinical case is presented in Figure 9.27.

For the placement of Z-Systems Z-Look3 Evo implants, the surgical protocol uses a conventional flapped technique, although a flapless technique is not specifically contraindicated within the company literature. As an aside, many of the surgical instruments and drills provided in the Z-Systems kit are made from zirconia or a ceramic material known as alumina-toughened zirconia (ATZ) and appear white in color. After the flap has been elevated, the ideal implant

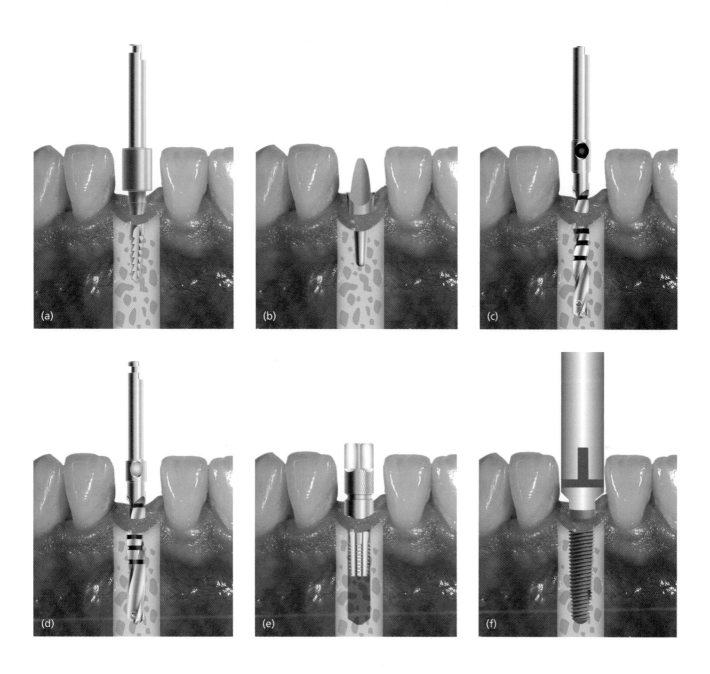

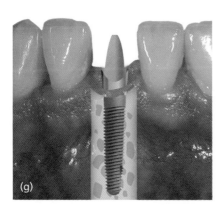

Figure 9.22 Zimmer One-Piece surgical protocol. (a) Pilot drill. (b) Try-in implant. (c) 2.3 mm twist drill. (d) 2.8/2.4 mm twist drill. (e) Bone tap (optional). (f) 3 mm diameter Zimmer One-Piece implant being placed with an implant driver, aligning the mark shown. (g) Zimmer One-Piece implant in place.

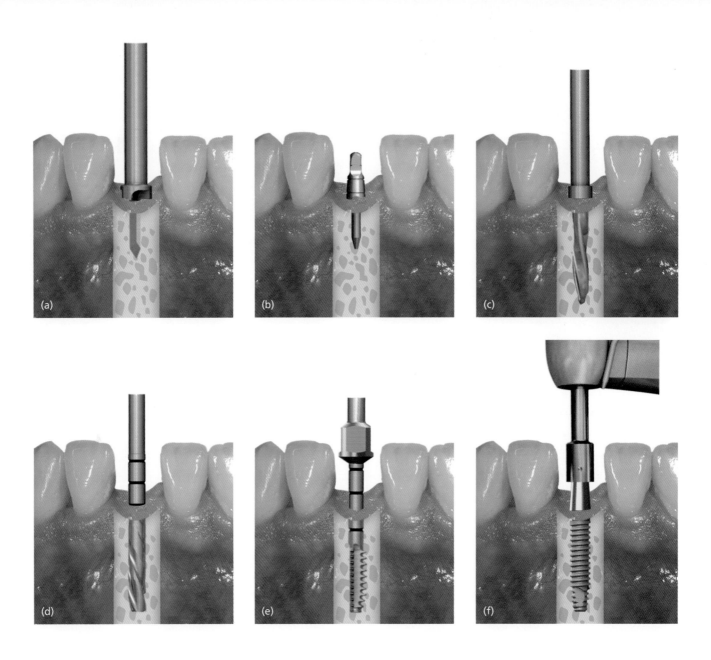

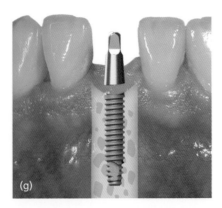

Figure 9.23 BioHorizons One-Piece 3.0 surgical protocol. (a) Alignment drill. (b) Trial implant. (c) 2.0 mm drill with stop. (d) 2.5 mm drill for type I bone (optional). (e) Bone tap (optional). (f) BioHorizons One Piece 3.0 implant being inserted with an implant driver. (g) BioHorizons One-Piece 3.0 implant in place.

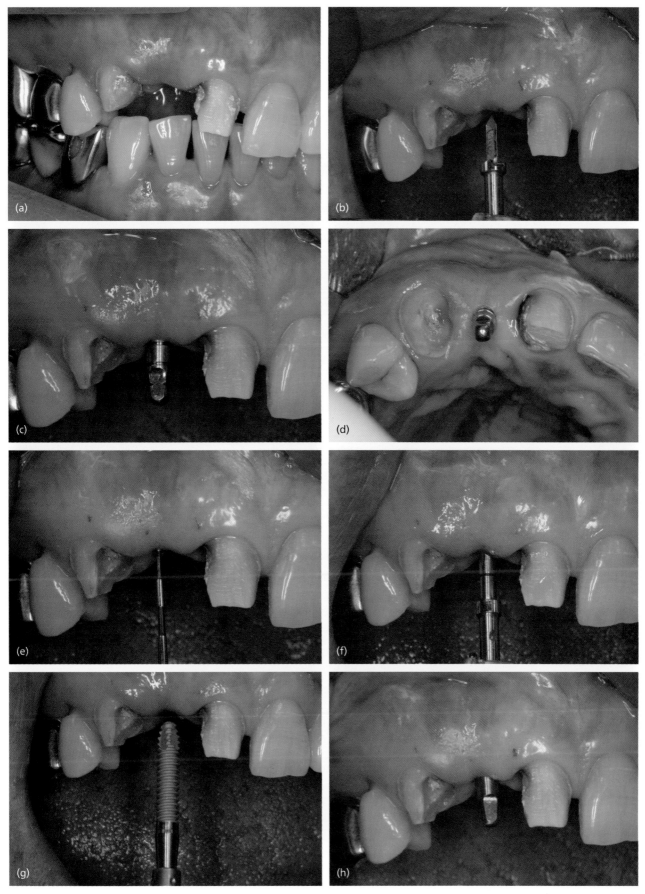

Figure 9.24 Placement and restoration of a BioHorizons One-Piece 3.0 implant. (a) Preoperative condition demonstrating missing tooth no. 7. The crowns for teeth no. 6 and no. 8 have been removed. (b) Alignment drill. (c) Try-in implant in place from frontal view. (d) Try-in implant in place from occlusal view; note the excellent mesiodistal and buccopalatal angulation. (e) Perio probe being used to assess soft tissue thickness. (f) 2.0 mm drill with stop creating proper depth of the osteotomy. (g) Implant being placed. (h) BioHorizons One Piece 3.0 implant in its final position after placement.

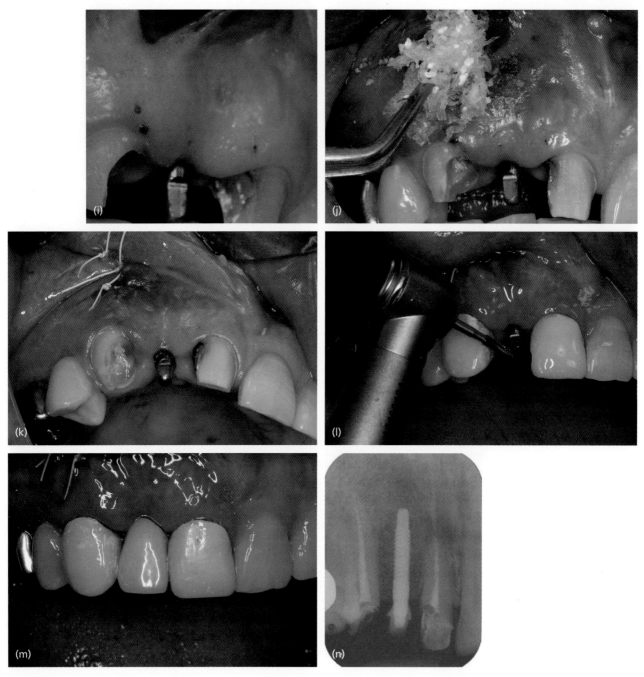

Figure 9.24 (*Continued*) (i) Vestibular incision used to examine the apical area of the implant, which was exposed through the buccal cortex. (j) Guided bone regeneration technique used to graft over the exposed implant surface. (k) Closure of the vestibular incision. (l) Preliminary adjustment of the abutment to accommodate the provisional restoration. (m) Provisional crowns over the implant at site no. 7 and teeth no. 6 and no. 8. (n) Postoperative radiograph showing excellent implant positioning.

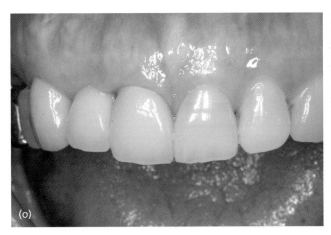
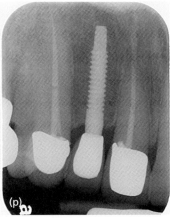

Figure 9.24 (*Continued*) (o) Final restoration of the implant at site no. 7 and with final PFM crowns for teeth no. 6 and no. 8. (p) Radiograph of the site after final restoration of the implant and adjacent teeth. Courtesy of Professor Dong-Seok Sohn, Catholic University Hospital of Daegu, Daegu, Republic of Korea.

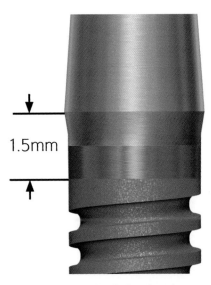

1.5mm

Figure 9.25 Appropriate depth for the placement of a BioHorizons One-Piece 3.0 implant.

location on the alveolar ridge is first marked with a 2.3 mm diameter round bur, and the initial osteotomy is then created at that location with a 2.3 mm diameter twist drill to the planned implant depth. It should be noted that the pointed tip of the implant drill (the *y* factor) is not accounted for within the depth lines along the bur and will add an additional 1.3 mm to the osteotomy depth. As an example, if the bur is inserted to the 6 mm depth line (the first line encountered), the actual osteotomy is 7.3 mm in depth.

After the initial osteotomy is created, the depth gauge should be used to examine the axis of the osteotomy to ensure proper angulation of the future implant. The osteotomy is then widened with subse-

quent twist drills until the drill corresponding to the planned implant width is reached. For 3.6 mm diameter implants, the last twist drill to be used is 2.85 mm in diameter. For 4.0 and 5.0 mm diameter implants, the last twist drills to be used are 3.25 and 3.75 mm in diameter, respectively. At this point in the procedure, the clinician must decide whether or not a countersink will need to be used on the crestal bone.

For the Z-Look3 Evo implants, a countersink is only to be used when the crestal bone is highly uneven and requires flattening. In the older surgical protocol for Z-Look3 implants, the shoulder had a variable insertion depth and the implant shoulder was often sunk up to 1.5 mm in the bone. The most current surgical protocol indicates that the shoulder of the Z-Look3 Evo implant should not be sunk more than 0.5 mm.

The next decision in the surgical protocol is whether or not to use a bone tap in the osteotomy. If the site is graded as type I bone (all cortical bone), the bone tap should be used along the entire length of the osteotomy. For type II bone with very firm crestal cortical bone, a bone tap can be used through the crestal cortical plate. For type III and IV bone, no tapping is indicated. The implant can then be placed using either a hand ratchet or handpiece. An insertion torque of at least 20 N-cm should be achieved upon implant placement, and torque values greater than 35 N-cm should be avoided according to company literature. The implant shoulder should be placed at approximately the level of the soft tissue or up to 1 mm below.

Bredent WhiteSKY Surgical Protocol

Bredent's surgical protocol for their whiteSKY implants is based upon attaining appropriate primary implant stability in all four bone quality types (Bredent 2011).

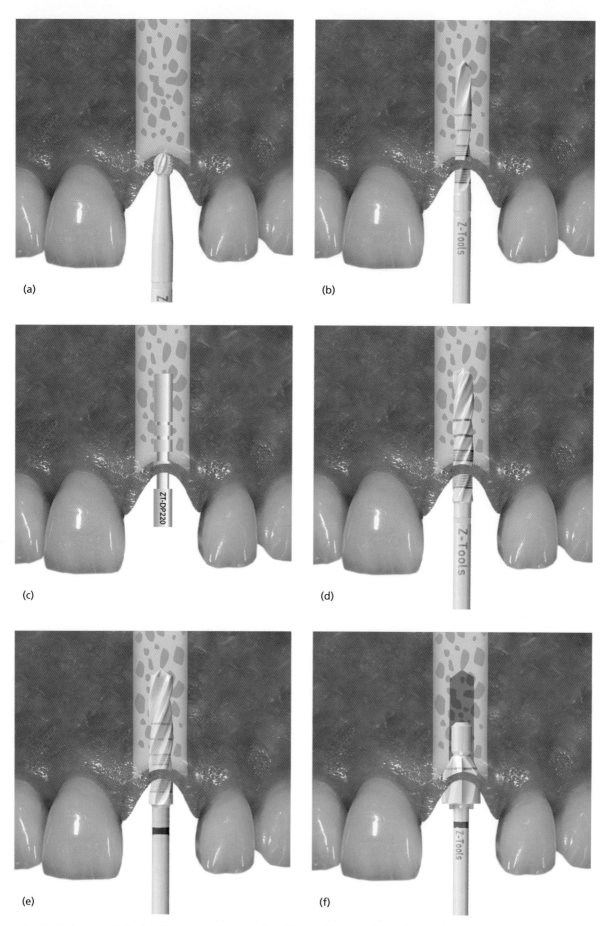

Figure 9.26 Z-Systems Z-Look3 Evo surgical protocol. (a) Round bur marking the ideal implant location. (b) 2.3 mm twist drill. (d) Depth gauge. (d) 2.85 mm twist drill. (e) 3.25 mm twist drill. (f) 4 mm countersink (optional).

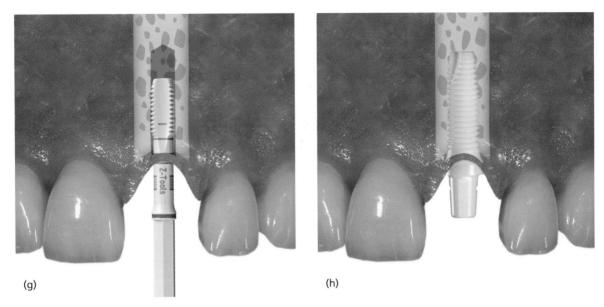

(g)   (h)

Figure 9.26   (Continued) (g) Bone tap (optional). (h) Z-Systems Z-Look3 Evo 4 × 11.5 mm implant inserted.

When using a flapped approach, a papilla-sparing incision design is recommended. Bredent does not indicate in the company literature whether or not a flapless technique is contraindicated for the whiteSKY implant. The initial drill to be used is a tapered pilot drill, which features a sharp tip to prevent slippage. It is to be used to its full 9 mm depth, and has an aggressive cutting surface at its most coronal 3 mm, which serves to prepare the cortical bone to a 3 mm diameter much like a countersink (Figure 9.28).

Preparing the cortical bone during the initial osteotomy is meant to spare the remaining drills from excessive use and allow proper angulation to be established more easily. The next step is to use a 2.25 mm diameter twist drill to the planned implant depth plus an additional 0.5 mm. Therefore, if a 10 mm implant is to be used, the twist drill should be used to a 10.5 mm depth. This additional necessary depth should be accounted for when determining the implant size to be used to avoid encroaching on nearby vital structures. Detachable drill stops are available to assist in attaining optimal depth. During this twist drill step, close attention should be paid to the buccolingual and mesiodistal angulation of the osteotomy being established.

At this point, the clinician must determine the bone quality at the osteotomy site in order to establish which family of drills to proceed with. For hard bone quality (type I–II), the "hard bone" drill set should be used in order of ascending diameter. For a 3.5 mm diameter implant, the 3.5 mm "hard bone" drill will be the final drill used to depth. If a wider implant is required, the clinician proceeds on to the 4.0 or 4.5 mm diameter drills as appropriate. If the bone quality is found to be soft (type III–IV), the "soft bone" drill set is used in the same manner based on the final implant diameter to be used.

The final preparation step is to use the crestal drill that corresponds to the planned implant diameter. These drills appear similar to the countersinks found in other surgical kits, and serve to properly prepare the coronal third of the site to match the conical–cylindrical hybrid shape of the implant. At this stage the site is ready for implant placement.

The implant may be placed with either the motorized handpiece or a hand ratchet. Primary stability is essential; the final implant torque should be between 20 and 45 N-cm for successful osseointegration. If a torque of 20 N-cm cannot be achieved, the implant should be removed and either a two-piece titanium implant placed or the site should be grafted for placement at a later date. If a torque of greater than 45 N-cm is achieved, the implant should be removed and the osteotomy widened slightly to decrease the risk of pressure necrosis of the adjacent bone.

The proper depth of implant placement is to the coronal edge of the sand-blasted portion of the implant. The stated length of the implant is from the apex to the edge of the sand-blasted surface. This measurement corresponds to the length displayed on the implant's packaging.

Figure 9.29 represents a clinical case where a Bredent whiteSKY implant is placed and restored.

Oral Iceberg CeraRoot Surgical Protocol

Oral Iceberg produces CeraRoot implants with five different designs created for replacement of specific

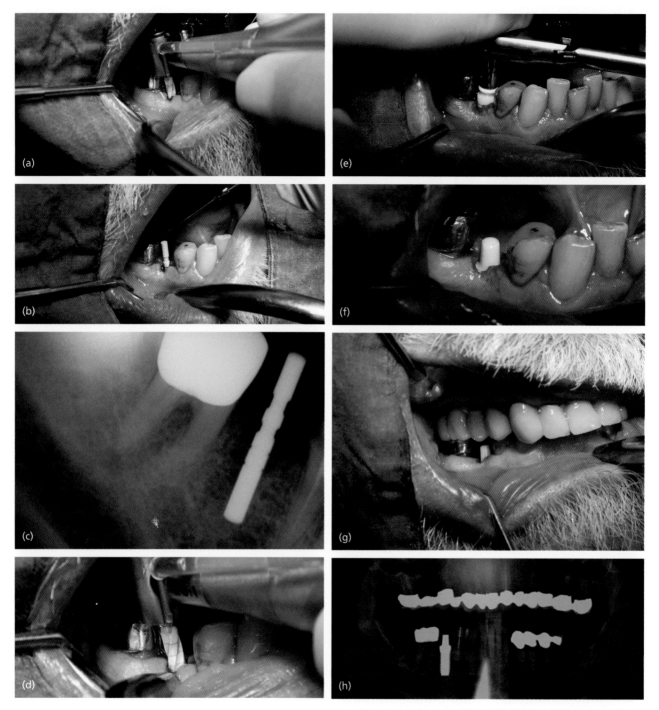

Figure 9.27 Placement of a Z-Systems Z-Look3 Evo implant. (a) Initial osteotomy being developed with a flapless technique. (b) Positioning pin in use. (c) Radiograph of positioning pin in place. (d) Final preparation of osteotomy. (e) Implant being placed with an implant driver and hand ratchet. (f) Implant in place. (g) Implant abutment with adequate clearance from maxillary dentition. (h) Radiograph of the implant after placement on the day of surgery. Courtesy of Z-Systems and Dr Martin Chares, Berlin, Germany.

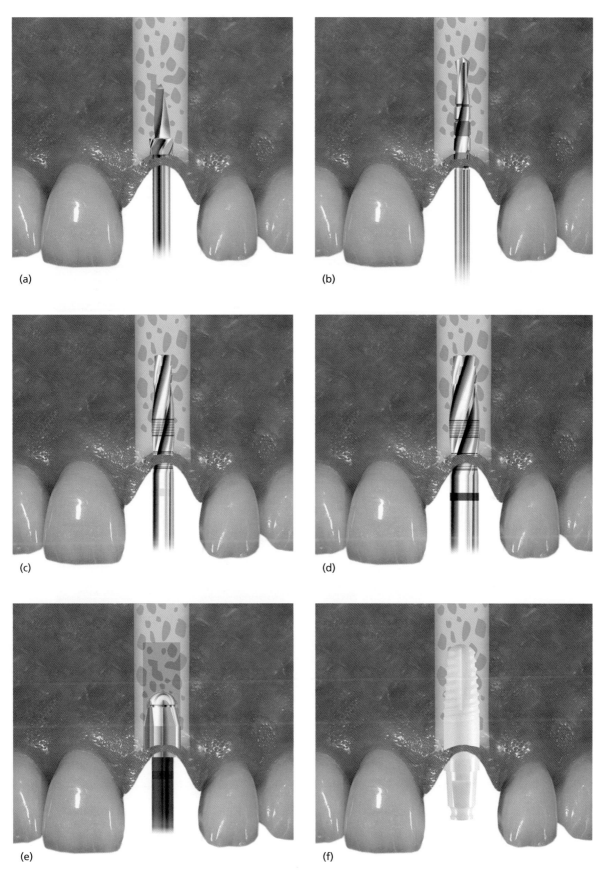

Figure 9.28 Bredent whiteSKY surgical protocol for a 4 × 12 mm implant in type I–II bone. (a) Tapered pilot drill. (b) 2.25 mm twist drill. (c) 3.5 mm "hard bone" drill. (d) 4.0 mm "hard bone" drill. (e) 4 mm crestal drill. (f) Bredent whiteSKY 4.0 × 12 mm implant inserted.

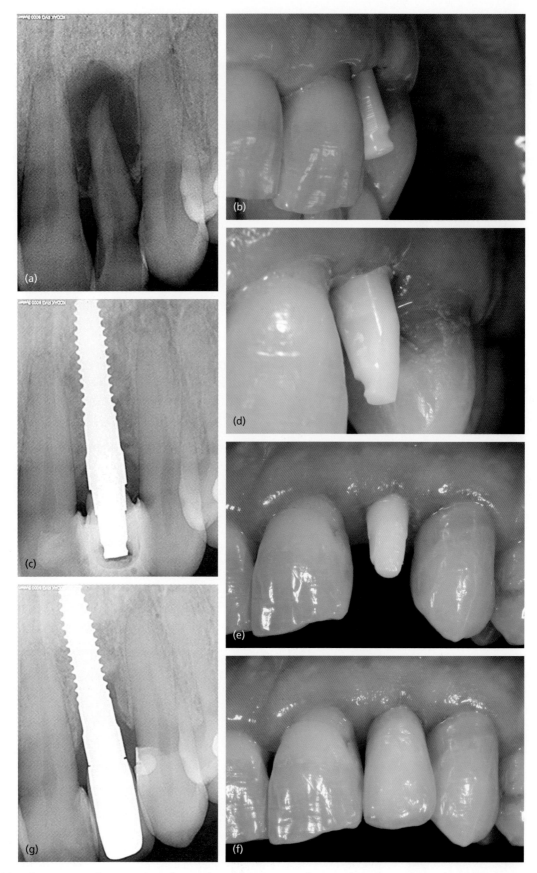

Figure 9.29 Placement and restoration of a Bredent whiteSKY implant. (a) Pre-extraction radiograph showing a large peri-apical radiolucency and hopeless prognosis. The tooth was subsequently extracted and a bone graft placed. (b) Initial positioning of the implant after placement. (c) Radiograph immediately post-implant placement and provisionalization. (d, e) Following final preparation of the abutment portion of the implant after healing and osseointegration. (f) Final restoration. (g) Radiograph of the final restoration. Courtesy of Dr Bernd Siewert, Clínica Somosaguas, Madrid, Spain.

teeth, each requiring a slightly different surgical protocol (Oral Iceberg 2009, 2012). A sample surgical protocol for one implant design is illustrated in Figure 9.30.

CeraRoot produces a "master kit" containing all the instruments necessary for th eplacement of all of their implant designs, as well as "starter kits" for each design containing only the instruments necessary for placement of that specific design. The instruments unique to each design are color coded to allow for ease of identification. CeraRoot does not indicate in their literature whether or not a flapless technique is contraindicated for their surgical protocol. They do, however, support the use of immediate implant placement when there is adequate bone volume and no active infection in the surgical site, provided that good primary stability can be achieved. Additionally, they recommend the use of a surgical guide for every case.

The surgical procedure begins with the use of a pointed pilot drill for development of the initial osteotomy to the planned implant depth. The osteotomy is then sequentially widened with 2.3, 2.8, and 3.5 mm twist drills. This will be the final osteotomy diameter when CeraRoot 12, 14, and 21 implants are to be used. Since the CeraRoot 12 is a parallel-walled implant, no further augmentation of the osteotomy is necessary. For the CeraRoot 14 and 21 implants, the corresponding countersink must be used prior to placement to widen the most coronal aspect of the osteotomy. For the CeraRoot 11 and 16 implants, the osteotomy must be further widened with the 4.2 mm twist drill and then prepared with the implant-specific countersink prior to implant placement.

When ready for placement, the implant is carried to the site with a plastic carrier that is attached to the implant when removed from its packaging. This transfer carrier is used to provide the initial stabilization of the implant in the osteotomy, and for all implants except the CeraRoot 14, the carrier can rotate the implant into the site until an instrument with greater torque is required. At this point, the titanium implant-specific driver from the surgical kit is used with either a torque wrench or handpiece to fully drive the implant into the site. The implant should be positioned such that the entire threaded portion of the implant is seated within bone. The implant must also be orientated such that the buccolingual and mesiodistal aspects of the implant are appropriately orientated within the arch, as each implant has a scalloped finish line and pre-prepared abutment that mimics the future tooth shape. Although the implant driver conceals the abutment portion of the implant during placement, there is a marking on the instrument that demonstrates the mid-buccal area to help with alignment. The transporter can also be momentarily removed to allow for direct visualization.

A clinical case demonstrating the placement and restoration of a CeraRoot 21 implant is presented in Figure 9.31.

The CeraRoot 14 implant requires a press-fit technique for placement. After the osteotomy is widened to 3.5 mm with twist drills to the planned depth, the site is prepared with the countersink. Since the cross-section of the implant at the crestal area has an ovoid shape, the osteotomy must be altered slightly to accommodate it. The countersink, after being used in the normal manner, is tipped slightly buccally and lingually within the site to create this ovoid shape. The CeraRoot 14 implant can then be carried to the site with the plastic transfer. Its buccolingual and mesiodistal aspects should be orientated appropriately from the time it is initially placed into the site, as there is no option for realignment once it has been placed. The implant is gently tapped into place with the inserting instrument and mallet to the desired depth.

ONE-PIECE IMPLANT ABUTMENT PREPARATION TECHNIQUES

The abutment portion of the implant often requires preparation in two phases (Figure 9.32).

Preliminary preparation may be required immediately following implant placement to ensure the abutment does not interfere with the occlusion and to accommodate the provisional restoration. The final preparation should only be completed after soft tissue healing and immediately prior to fabrication of the final restoration. Preparation of the abutment surface can potentially generate excessive heat in the implant and surrounding bone, particularly with titanium one-piece implants (Cohen et al. 2010). To minimize this possibility, the burs should be used at 200,000–280,000 rpm and pressed lightly onto the abutment surface in short bursts. Burs should be replaced frequently to maintain cutting efficiency. Copious saline irrigation should be utilized at all times during preparation to help dissipate the heat produced and minimize any adverse effects on the adjacent bone (Gabay et al. 2010). A minimum irrigation of 50 ml/min is recommended for both zirconia and titanium abutment preparation. Specialized kits are available for the preparation of both titanium and zirconia (Figure 9.33), and it is imperative to use the correct burs as their cutting efficiency will minimize the total working time needed and the potential for excessive heat generation.

In general, titanium abutments should be initially prepared with carbide burs with aggressive cutting blades and then finished with finishing carbide burs.

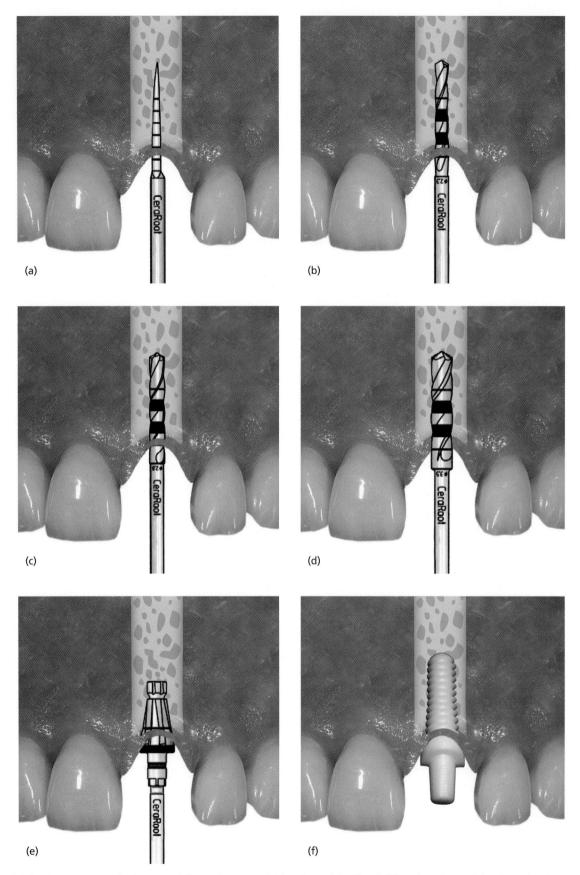

Figure 9.30 CeraRoot surgical protocol for a CeraRoot 21 implant. (a) Pilot drill to the planned implant depth. (b) 2.3 mm twist drill. (c) 2.8 mm twist drill. (d) 3.5 mm twist drill. (e) CeraRoot 21 countersink. (f) CeraRoot 21 implant in place.

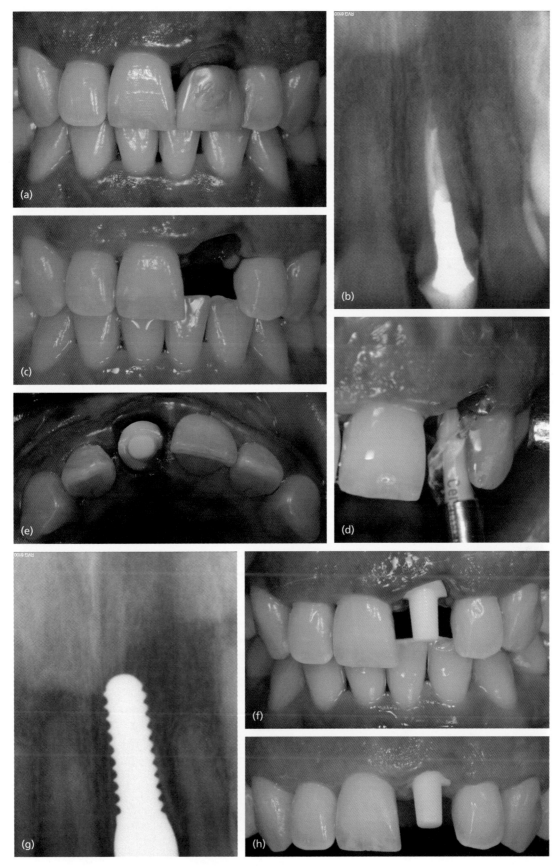

Figure 9.31 Placement and restoration of a CeraRoot 21 implant. (a) Preoperative clinical appearance of tooth no. 9. (b) Preoperative radiograph. (c) Following an atraumatic extraction of tooth no. 9. (d) Preparation of the osteotomy for immediate implant placement. (e) Occlusal view of the implant immediately after implant insertion. (f) Frontal view of the implant immediately following implant insertion. (g) Radiograph immediately following implant insertion.

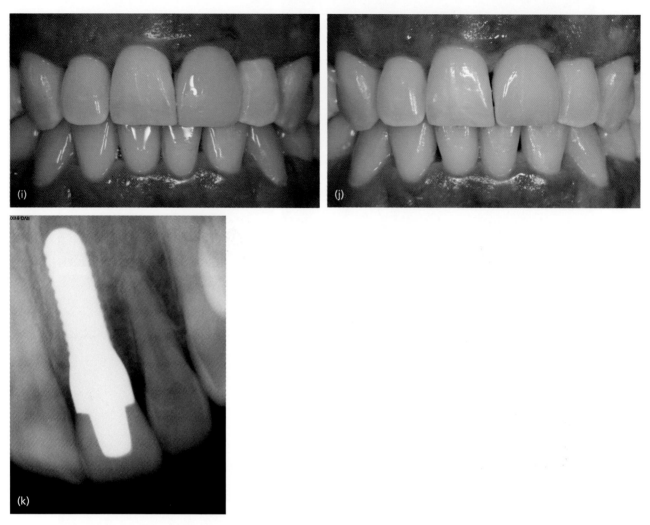

Figure 9.31 (*Continued*) (h) After 4 months of soft tissue healing. (i) With a provisional crown over the implant at site no. 9. (j) Final restoration of the implant at site no. 9. (k) Radiograph of the final restoration. Courtesy of Oral Iceberg.

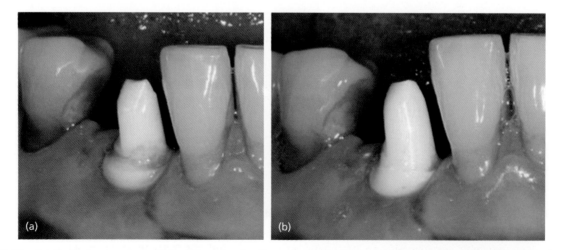

Figure 9.32 (a) Preliminary preparation. Sort tissue healing occurred prior to final preparation. The abutment height was lowered to create room for a provisional restoration, but the finish line was not contoured. (b) Final preparation just prior to impression taking. Note that the sharp corners have been removed, the abutment angulation has been adjusted, and the finish line has been contoured. Courtesy of Z-Systems.

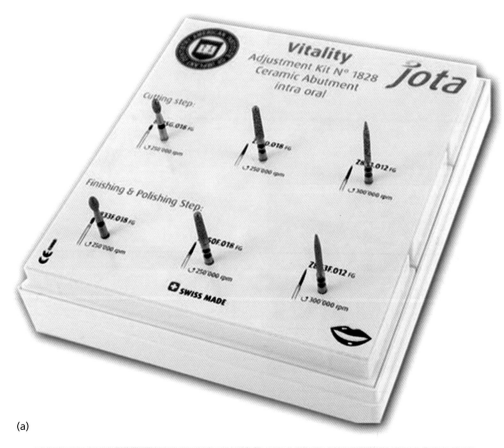

(a)

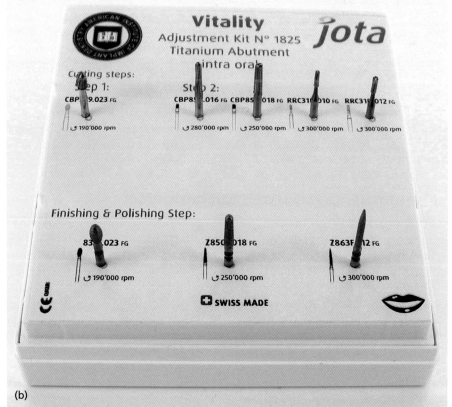

(b)

Figure 9.33 Examples of adjustment kits made specifically for titanium and zirconia. (a) Zirconia adjustment kit containing blue- and red-ring diamond burs. (b) Titanium adjustment kit containing the appropriate carbide burs. Courtesy of Jota.

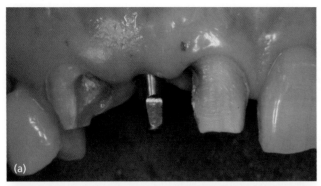

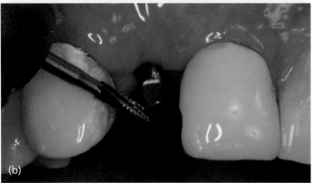

Figure 9.34 (a) Appearance of the abutment portion of a one-piece implant immediately following placement. (b) Preliminary preparation of the abutment, including lowering the abutment height in order to accommodate the planned provisional restoration. Courtesy of Professor Dong-Seok Sohn, Catholic University Hospital of Daegu, Daegu, Republic of Korea.

The gross reduction of zirconia abutments should be with blue-ring diamond burs (120 microns) and the finishing steps accomplished with red ring (47 microns) diamond burs. For the most complete description of the specific burs required, see Chapter 8.

Preliminary Adjustments

It is not recommended to prepare the implant for the final restoration during preliminary adjustments on the day of implant placement. Only the adjustments necessary to accommodate the planned type of provisional should be completed. Often the abutment height needs to be decreased so the abutment will not interfere with the occlusion and the provisional restoration will have an adequate thickness (Figure 9.34).

Additionally, the abutment portion may require some amount of angulation for proper alignment. When any amount of preparation is required, a rubber dam should always be used to minimize the possibility of debris being forced into the surgical site.

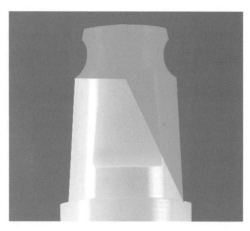

Figure 9.35 Abutment shape following final preparation compared with the unaltered abutment. Note that the abutment height has been lowered and the abutment has been angulated, but enough height of abutment remains to create retention for the future restoration. Courtesy of Bredent.

Final Adjustments

After the appropriate healing period and when osseointegration has been verified, the final preparation can be completed (Figure 9.35).

The adjustments commonly needed are abutment height reduction, finish line contouring, angulation, and occasionally the addition of retentive features. The abutment height should be at least 2 mm below the occlusal plane to provide for adequate bulk of restorative material. Excessive height reduction should be avoided as it will compromise retention form. Generally, the required abutment height is thought to be at least one-third of the definitive crown height for appropriate retention.

Finish Line

For NobelDirect and BioHorizons 3.0 mm diameter implants, no specific finish line is recommended in the company literature. It has been published that a knife-edge margin should be used for 3.0 mm diameter implants, as a chamfer margin may compromise the structure of the already narrow implant (Sohn et al. 2011). Based on the authors' experience, the most esthetic outcomes are achieved with chamfer margins owing to the fact that a porcelain margin can be used. With NobelDirect and BioHorizons 3.0 mm diameter implants, either a knife edge or a light chamfer margin (not exceeding 0.25 mm in axial depth) can be used. However, esthetics might be less than ideal since these designs do not allow for a porcelain margin. An

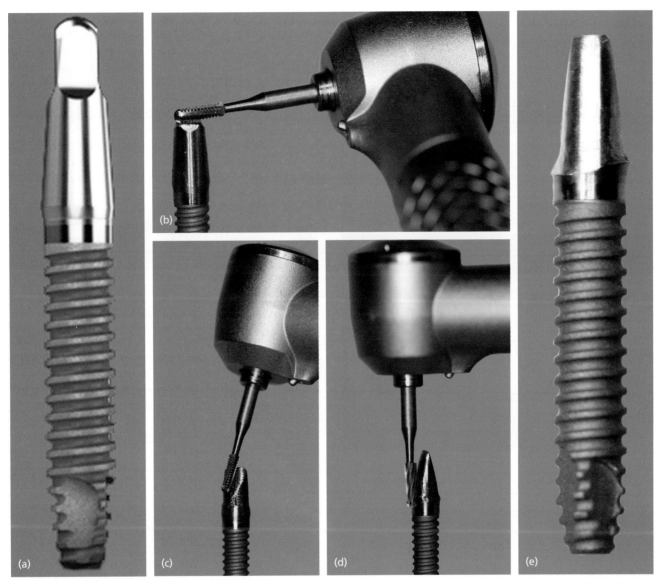

Figure 9.36 Preparation of the abutment portion of a BioHorizons One-Piece 3.0 implant. (a) Unaltered implant. (b) Reduction of abutment height using a carbide bur with aggressive cutting blades. (c) Margin preparation and angulation of the abutment using a carbide bur with aggressive cutting blades. (d) Finishing the preparation with a finishing carbide bur. (e) Final abutment preparation with a tapered shape and light chamfer margin after finishing.

example preparation of a BioHorizons implant is presented in Figure 9.36.

If esthetics are of great concern, one might consider using a Zimmer One-Piece implant as a prepared chamfer margin is an intrinsic feature. The Zimmer One-Piece prepared margin should obviate the need for margin preparation, although the facial margin may need adjusting if it remains supragingival after soft tissue healing. When the wider one-piece Nobel-Direct implants are used, a chamfer margin should be prepared at a 0.5 mm subgingival position with a 0.5 mm axial depth.

Each of the three zirconia implant designs discussed in this chapter has a prepared finish line as an intrinsic feature. The Z-Systems Z-Look3 Evo and Bredent whiteSKY designs have flat finish lines and may require minor adjustments if the margin remains supragingival after the healing phase to attain the appropriate subgingival position. The Oral Iceberg Ceraroot implants, on the other hand, are designed with anatomic shapes and scalloped finish lines, in order to minimize the amount of preparation necessary.

Often, however, the soft tissue response to the Zirconia surface causes an overgrowth of gingival

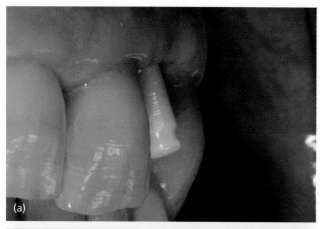

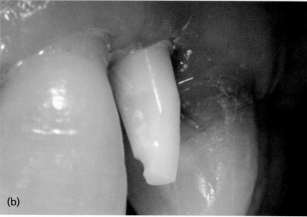

Figure 9.37   (a) Unadjusted abutment demonstrating a slight buccal angulation. (b) Excellent angulation of the abutment achieved after preparation, which will allow for adequate space for the restoration. Courtesy of Dr Bernd Siewert, Clínica Somosaguas, Madrid, Spain.

tissue and an uncovering procedure with a scalpel or electrocautery may be required to expose the finish line if a provisional crown is not closely adapted during healing.

Abutment Angulation

Angulation of the abutment should be completed when necessary to allow for the proper trajectory of the crown and an adequate amount of space for restorative material along the facial surface (Figure 9.37).

For narrow-diameter implants in the esthetic zone, the abutment should align with the adjacent incisal edges. For implants used in other sites, the abutment should align with the central fossae of the adjacent teeth. For the titanium one-piece implants, company literature for NobelDirect and BioHorizons indicates that the abutment should not be angled more than 10 degrees from the long axis of the implant. Zimmer One-Piece implants are manufactured with both

straight and 17-degree angled abutments; deciding which to use should ideally be planned preoperatively. Zimmer advises against all but the minimum preparation of the titanium surface, and preparation can be minimized by choosing the appropriate implant.

For the zirconia one-piece implants, Z-Systems indicates that an angulation of the abutment up to 20 degrees is acceptable for their Z-Look3 Evo implants, while Bredent whiteSKY and Oral Iceberg Ceraroot do not address this issue within their literature. Based on these recommendations, the authors believe an appropriate guideline is to limit abutment angulations to 20 degrees or less, and to carefully plan treatment so that greater angulations are not necessary. In situations where greater angulations will be required, one-piece implants are not appropriate.

Post-adjustment Smoothing

When all major adjustments have been completed, the preparation should be checked to ensure that no sharp edges or corners remain. For both titanium and zirconia one-piece implants, smoothing burs are often provided in the prefabricated adjustment kits and should be used for this purpose. For zirconia implants this step is especially important, as sharp areas could be prone to fracture and could potentially compromise the long-term stability of the implant.

PRINCIPLES OF LOADING

Determining how and when to load one-piece implants is a necessary part of treatment planning. As previously discussed, one-piece implants will always be subjected to some amount of loading from the time of placement onward. As most one-piece implant cases are also esthetic zone cases, there must be a balance between the need for esthetic-appearing provisional restorations and the reduction of forces placed on the implant. Immediate loading of titanium implants with advanced surface characteristics in the esthetic zone has been shown to be a predictably successful protocol (Mijiritsky et al. 2009; Tortamano et al. 2010; Den Hartog et al. 2011). As the titanium one-piece implant designs covered in this text all have advanced surface characteristics, they can be subjected to an immediate load protocol, although immediate function is not recommended. During the transition between primary and secondary stability, these implants can maintain cemented provisional crown restorations kept out of functional occlusion. The final restoration is generally placed after 2–6 months of provisionalization depending on operator preference and the presence of any

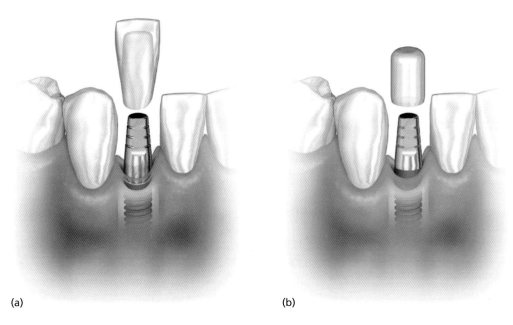

(a)   (b)

Figure 9.38 (a) Placement of an acrylic provisional crown over the abutment portion of a titanium one-piece implant. (b) Healing cap. This is an implant-specific plastic cap that fits precisely over the abutment portion of the unprepared one-piece implant. The healing cap can be bonded to the abutment as is or acrylic can be added to its surface to create an anatomic provisional crown. Courtesy of Nobel Biocare.

compromising factors such as concurrent bone grafting.

Zirconia one-piece implants, on the other hand, should be subjected to a protected loading protocol. Due to the surface characteristics of the designs covered in this chapter, the transition between primary and secondary stability takes an average of 6–8 weeks longer than implants with advanced surface characteristics. Clinically, this translates into a need to maximize the protection of the exposed abutment portion of the implant. Based on the authors' experience, this is best accomplished by the use of an Essix appliance, although other methods presented in company literature will be discussed in the following section. Following the period of protected loading, the implants are placed into functional occlusion in the range of 3–6 months post placement.

PROVISIONALIZATION AND CROWN FABRICATION

Provisional Restorations for Titanium One-piece Implants

As the titanium one-piece implants covered in this chapter can all support immediate loading, the primary method for provisionalization is a cemented temporary crown (Figure 9.38a).

There are many ways of making these provisional crowns. One method involves the chairside fabrication of an acrylic crown. This may be accomplished by placing acrylic in a thermoform tray or relining a shell crown. Another method involves the use of an implant-specific plastic healing cap (Figure 9.38b), which are manufactured by many companies. These healing caps are non-anatomic but closely fit the abutment surface, and the pre-established finish line, when present. If esthetics are not a concern, the healing cap can be left as is and cemented to the abutment. To create a more natural appearance, the healing cap may be placed inside a shell crown with a pick-up technique or acrylic can be added by hand to the outer portion of the healing cap to create an anatomic provisional crown. It should be noted, however, that when preliminary adjustments need to be made to the abutment, these temporary healing caps may not fit properly and cannot therefore be used. A laboratory-made provisional crown can also be requested preoperatively and relined or adjusted as necessary postoperatively.

Nobel Biocare recommends that temporary restoration margins are placed 0.5 mm supragingival during the healing phase. BioHorizons does not provide recommendations for margin placement. However, from traditional prosthodontics we know that margins closer than 2 mm to the crestal bone will impinge on the biologic width and incite chronic tissue inflammation in the area. Provisional restorations placed on

Zimmer implants should be well adapted to the finish line to prevent tissue ingrowth during healing.

These provisional restorations should be kept out of occlusion in centric position as well as during lateral excursive and protrusive movements. Functional loading during the healing period may compromise osseointegration. Once placed, removing the cemented provisional restoration is not recommended during the healing phase, as the torque required may adversely affect osseointegration.

Provisional Restorations for Zirconia One-piece Implants

For zirconia one-piece implants, the exposed abutment portion of the implant must have maximum protection during the healing phase. This is because secondary stability will be slower than for their titanium counterparts. Based on the authors' experience, the device that offers the best protection is the Essix appliance (Figure 9.39).

Tooth-colored composite or acrylic can be added to the implant site for esthetics as long as there is at least 1 mm of clearance between the abutment and the appliance in all dimensions during function. For posterior teeth where there is little esthetic concern, the tooth-colored material can be withheld, which allows for easy visualization of the amount of clearance provided. The device should be worn during eating and sleeping, and only removed for cleaning. This allows the maximum amount of protection from chewing forces, as well as from pressure from the tongue and cheek tissues.

There are many other methods mentioned throughout the literature that may also provide adequate protection for the zirconia one-piece implant. When the patient has an existing removable partial denture (RPD) with adequate stability and retention, this may be relieved to provide the appropriate clearance for the abutment. An interim laboratory-made RPD that has been relieved in the area of the implants can be used, which may be particularly useful when replacing multiple teeth in the esthetic zone (Figure 9.40).

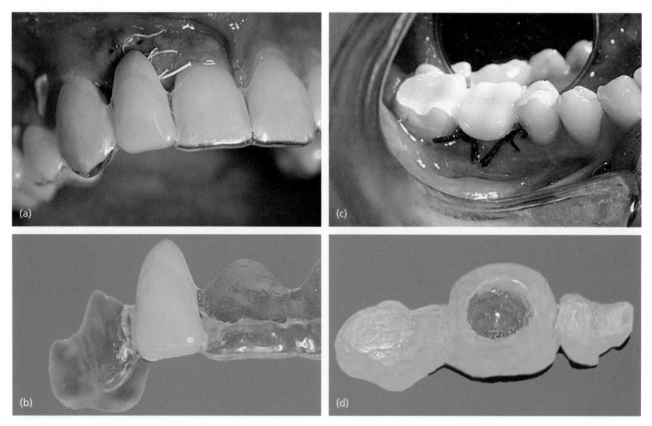

Figure 9.39 (a) Essix appliance in use as a provisional restoration for a zirconia one-piece implant. (b) Essix appliance. Note that the internal portion of the white acrylic has been removed to accommodate the abutment portion of the implant. (c) Alternative type of protective appliance for a zirconia one-piece implant: a fixed partial denture design utilizing inlay preparations on the adjacent teeth. (d) The fixed partial denture provisional restoration, where the internal portion of the pontic has been removed to accommodate the abutment portion of the one-piece implant. Courtesy of Bredent.

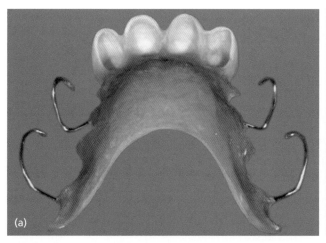
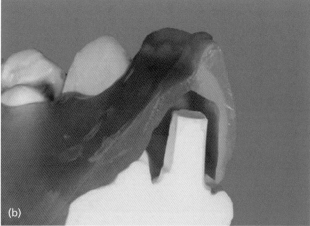

Figure 9.40 (a) Removable partial denture (RPD) design as a provisional restoration for one-piece zirconia implants. (b) RPD design demonstrating the clearance required to protect the one-piece zirconia abutments during the healing phase. Courtesy of Z-Systems/OralDesign Boden See.

When adjacent teeth are also being restored, a fixed partial denture design with no contact on the implant abutment can be used. This is best constructed from a reinforced resin (Figure 9.39c, d). Other options for fixed provisionals include constructing a fixed partial denture on temporary implants adjacent to the one-piece implant, or creating a ceramic Maryland bridge which is relieved in the area of the abutment. The drawback of these designs is that they do not adapt to the restorative finish line and cannot shape the gingiva during healing. An alternative method that allows for this is to cement a small provisional crown over the zirconia abutment, and to use a protective Essix appliance that does not contact the crown. Appliances should be checked periodically during the healing period to ensure adequate clearance, especially when tissue supported, as resolution of postoperative tissue swelling may affect fit.

Tissues often adapt very well to the zirconia surface and may cover the restorative finish line when the provisional device does not adapt to it. After an adequate amount of time for osseointegration has passed, which may be 3–6 months depending on multiple factors, the excess tissue may be excised and a cemented provisional crown can be fabricated to contour the gingiva prior to taking the final impression.

Cementation of Provisional Restorations

With any method that involves the use of cement, a postoperative radiograph should be taken to insure no excess cement has been trapped within the sulcus. Cement left after provisional placement can be highly irritating to the healing soft tissues and may compromise the final esthetic outcome.

Final Impression

When ready for the final restoration, the provisional one should be removed and any final preparation of the abutment completed, as described previously. The final impression can be taken in a manner similar that of conventional crown and bridge therapy. A retraction cord can be placed prior to the impression to allow for a subgingival margin to be created in the final restoration. Polyvinylsiloxane is the impression material of choice for these cases. Light body material can be syringed into the sulcus area and around the abutment and adjacent teeth, while regular body material can be placed in the impression tray.

The final impression must capture the margin circumferentially to be appropriate for use. Some companies manufacture prefabricated impression caps that can be placed over the abutments and picked up within the elastomeric impression material. These are advantageous in that they precisely capture the restorative margin and eliminate the need for a retraction cord. However, in cases where adjustment of the margin is necessary, they cannot be used. CAD/CAM digital impressions are also being used as an alternative to the traditional final impression.

Final Prosthesis

Final prostheses should be manufactured to allow for the best esthetic result while minimizing deleterious forces on the implant restoration. Final restorations for the titanium one-piece implants should be PFM designs (Figure 9.41).

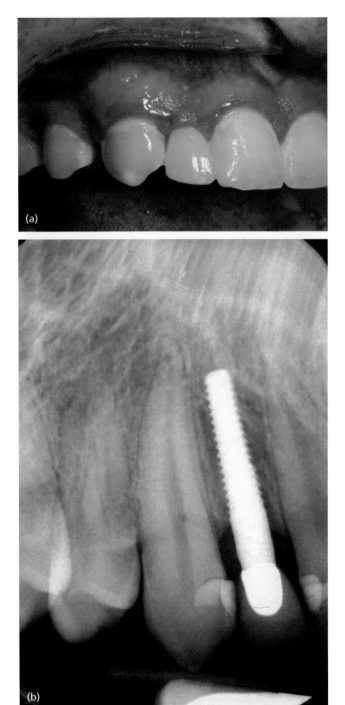

Figure 9.41 (a) Final restoration using a Nobel Biocare NobelDirect one-piece implant at the maxillary lateral incisor site. (b) Radiograph taken after delivery of the final restoration. Courtesy of Dr Stephen M. Parel, DDS.

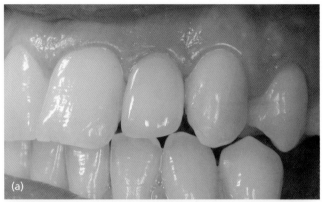

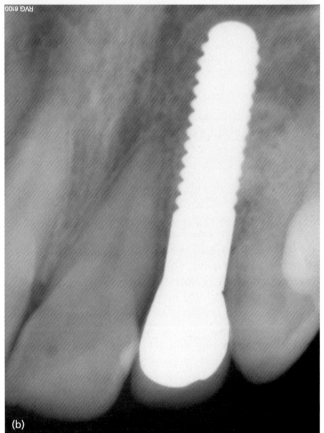

Figure 9.42 (a) Final restoration using an Oral Iceberg CeraRoot one-piece implant at the maxillary lateral incisor site. (b) Radiograph taken after delivery of the final restoration. Courtesy of Oral Iceberg.

Zirconia one-piece implants, on the other hand, should be restored with all-ceramic crowns, preferably with zirconia copings (Figure 9.42).

The implants should be placed into function such that loads are placed along the long axis of the implant, while lateral forces are minimized. The margin should be checked for appropriate fit. In esthetic zone cases, margins can be placed up to 1 mm subgingival. The final restoration should be cemented with soft-access cement, and a final radiograph should be taken to confirm removal of all the cement from the sulcus.

REFERENCES AND ADDITIONAL READING

Allum, S.R., Tomlinson, R.A., & Joshi, R. (2008). The impact of loads on standard diameter, small diameter and mini implants: a comparative laboratory study. *Clinical Oral Implants Research*, 19(6), 553–559.

Atieh, M.A., Payne, A.G., Duncan, W.J., De Silva, R.K., & Cullinan, M.P. (2010). Immediate placement or immediate restoration/loading of single implants for molar tooth replacement: a systematic review and meta-analysis. *International Journal of Oral and Maxillofacial Implants*, 25(2), 401–415.

BioHorizons (2010). *BioHorizons Procedure Manual ML0109*. BioHorizons, USA.

Borgonovo, A.E., Arnaboldi, O., Censi, R., Dolci, M., & Santoro, G. (2010). Edentulous jaws rehabilitation with yttrium-stabilized zirconium dioxide implants: two years follow-up experience. *Minerva Stomatologica*, 59(7/8), 381–392.

Bredent (2011). *Bredent whiteSKY Procedure Manual 426 GB 2*. Bredent Medical, Germany.

Cales, B. & Stefani, Y. (1994). Mechanical properties and surface analysis of retrieved zirconia hip joint heads after an implantation time of two to three years. *Journal of Materials Science*, 5(6/7), 376–380.

Cohen, O., Gabay, E., & Machtei, E.E. (2010). Cooling profile following prosthetic preparation of 1-piece dental implants. *Journal of Oral Implantology*, 36(4), 273–279.

Crespi, R., Capparé, P., Gherlone, E., & Romanos, G.E. (2008). Immediate versus delayed loading of dental implants placed in fresh extraction sockets in the maxillary esthetic zone: a clinical comparative study. *International Journal of Oral and Maxillofacial Implants*, 23(4), 753–758.

Den Hartog, L., Raghoebar, G.M., Stellingsma, K., Vissink, A., & Meijer, H.J. (2011). Immediate non-occlusal loading of single implants in the aesthetic zone: a randomized clinical trial. *Journal of Clinical Periodontology*, 38(2), 186–194.

Esposito, M., Grusovin, M.G., Willings, M., Coulthard, P., & Worthington, H.V. (2007). The effectiveness of immediate, early, and conventional loading of dental implants: a Cochrane systematic review of randomized controlled clinical trials. *International Journal of Oral and Maxillofacial Implants*, 22(6), 893–904.

Finne, K., Rompen, E., & Toljanic, J. (2007a). Clinical evaluation of a prospective multicenter study on 1-piece implants. Part 1: marginal bone level evaluation after 1 year of follow-up. *International Journal of Oral and Maxillofacial Implants*, 22(2), 226–234.

Finne, K., Rompen, E., & Toljanic, J. (2007b). Prospective multicenter study of marginal bone level and soft tissue health of a one-piece implant after two years. *Journal of Prosthetic Dentistry*, 97(Suppl 6), S79–85.

Froum, S.J., Cho, S.C., Elian, N., et al. (2011). Survival rate of one-piece dental implants placed with a flapless or flap protocol – a randomized, controlled study: 12-month results. *International Journal of Periodontics and Restorative Dentistry*, 31(6), 591–601.

Gabay, E., Cohen, O., & Machtei, E.E. (2010). Heat production during prosthetic preparation of a one-piece dental implant. *International Journal of Oral and Maxillofacial Implants*, 25(6), 1131–1136.

Glauser, R., Schüpbach, P., Gottlow, J., & Hämmerle, C.H. (2005). Periimplant soft tissue barrier at experimental one-piece mini-implants with different surface topography in humans: a light-microscopic overview and histometric analysis. *Clinical Implant Dentistry and Related Research*, 7(Suppl 1), S44–51.

Glauser, R., Zembic, A., Ruhstaller, P., & Windisch, S. (2007). Five-year results of implants with an oxidized surface placed predominantly in soft quality bone and subjected to immediate occlusal loading. *Journal of Prosthetic Dentistry*, 97(Suppl 6), S59–68.

Hahn, J.A. (2007). Clinical and radiographic evaluation of one-piece implants used for immediate function. *Journal of Oral Implantology*, 33(3), 152–155.

Hermann, J.S., Buser, D., Schenk, R.K., Schoolfield, J.D., & Cochran, D.L. (2001). Biologic width around one- and two-piece titanium implants. *Clinical Oral Implants Research*, 12(6), 559–571.

Jivraj, S., Reshad, M., & Chee, W.W. (2005). Critical appraisal. Immediate loading of implants in the esthetic zone. *Journal of Esthetic and Restorative Dentistry*, 17(5), 320–325.

Koch, F.P., Weng, D., Krämer, S., Biesterfeld, S., Jahn-Eimermacher, A., & Wagner, W. (2010). Osseointegration of one-piece zirconia implants compared with a titanium implant of identical design: a histomorphometric study in the dog. *Clinical Oral Implants Research*, 21(3), 350–356.

Kohal, R.J., Papavasiliou, G., Kamposiora, P., Tripodakis, A., & Strub, J.R. (2002). Three-dimensional computerized stress analysis of commercially pure titanium and yttrium-partially stabilized zirconia implants. *International Journal of Prosthodontics*, 15(2), 189–194.

Kohal, R.J., Wolkewitz, M., & Tsakona, A. (2011). The effects of cyclic loading and preparation on the fracture strength of zirconium-dioxide implants: an in vitro investigation. *Clinical Oral Implants Research*, 22(8), 808–814.

Mijiritsky, E., Mardinger, O., Mazor, Z., & Chaushu, G. (2009). Immediate provisionalization of single-tooth implants in fresh-extraction sites at the maxillary esthetic zone: up to 6 years of follow-up. *Implant Dentistry*, 18(4), 326–333.

Nasatzky, E., Gultchin, J., & Schwartz, Z. (2003). [The role of surface roughness in promoting osteointegration.] *Refuat Hapeh Vehashinayim*, 20(3), 8–19, 98.

Nobel Biocare (2005). *NobelDirect Clinical Procedure and Product Catalog 9643, GB 0505*. Nobel Biocare AB, Switzerland.

Oliva, J., Oliva, X., & Oliva, J.D. (2007). One-year follow-up of first consecutive 100 zirconia dental implants in humans: a comparison of 2 different rough surfaces. *International Journal of Oral and Maxillofacial Implants*, 22(3), 430–435.

Oliva, J., Oliva, X., & Oliva, J.D. (2010). Five-year success rate of 831 consecutively placed zirconia dental implants in humans: a comparison of three different rough surfaces. *International Journal of Oral and Maxillofacial Implants*, 25(2), 336–344.

Oral Iceberg (2009). *CeraRoot Procedure Manual W055*. Oral Iceberg, Spain.

Oral Iceberg (2012). *CeraRoot Procedure Manual 009.150*. Oral Iceberg, Spain.

Osathanon, T., Bespinyowong, K., Arksornnukit, M., Takahashi, H., & Pavasant, P. (2011). Human osteoblast-like cell spreading and proliferation on Ti-6Al-7Nb surfaces of varying roughness. *Journal of Oral Science*, 53(1), 23–30.

Parel, S.M. & Schow, S.R. (2005). Early clinical experience with a new one-piece implant system in single tooth sites. *Journal of Oral and Maxillofacial Surgery* 63(9 Suppl 2), 2–10.

Reddy, M.S., O'Neal, S.J., Haigh, S., Aponte-Wesson, R., & Geurs, N.C. (2008). Initial clinical efficacy of 3-mm implants immediately placed into function in conditions of limited spacing. *International Journal of Oral and Maxillofacial Implants*, 23(2), 281–288.

Scarano, A., Piattelli, M., Caputi, S., Favero, G.A., & Piattelli, A. (2004). Bacterial adhesion on commercially pure titanium and zirconium oxide disks: an in vivo human study. *Journal of Periodontology*, 75(2), 292–296.

Schuepbach, P. & Glauser, R. (2012). TiUnite® – a unique biomaterial. *Nobel BioCare News*, June. http://newsletter.nobelbiocare.com/2012/06/tiunite-a-unique-biomaterial/print/ (last accessed April 2014).

Siepenkothen, T. (2007). Clinical performance and radiographic evaluation of a novel single-piece implant in a private practice over a mean of seventeen months. *Journal of Prosthetic Dentistry*, 97(Suppl 6), S69–78.

Siepenkothen, T., Cluader, A., & Mehlau, R. (2006). Multiple center clinical and radiographic evaluation of one-piece implants: a retrospective six-year evaluation. *European Journal of Oral Implantology*, 2(Suppl 1), 4–11.

Silva, N.R., Coelho, P.G., Fernandes, C.A., Navarro, J.M., Dias, R.A., & Thompson, V.P. (2009). Reliability of one-piece ceramic implant. *Journal of Biomedical Materials Research, B Applied Biomaterials*, 88(2), 419–426.

Sohn, D.S., Bae, M.S., Heo, J.U., Park, J.S., Yea, S.H., & Romanos, G.E. (2011). Retrospective multicenter analysis of immediate provisionalization using one-piece narrow-diameter (3.0-mm) implants. *International Journal of Oral and Maxillofacial Implants*, 26(1), 163–168.

Stadlinger, B., Hennig, M., Eckelt, U., Kuhlisch, E., & Mai, R. (2010). Comparison of zirconia and titanium implants after a short healing period. A pilot study in minipigs. *International Journal of Oral and Maxillofacial Surgery*, 39(6), 585–592.

Tortamano, P., Camargo, L.O., Bello-Silva, M.S., & Kanashiro, L.H. (2010). Immediate implant placement and restoration in the esthetic zone: a prospective study with 18 months of follow-up. *International Journal of Oral and Maxillofacial Implants*, 25(2), 345–350.

Zimmer Dental (2007). *Zimmer Dental Procedure Manual 7458A*. Zimmer Dental, USA.

Z-Systems (2008). *Z-Systems Surgical and Prosthetic Concept Manual*. Z-Systems, Switzerland.

10

Cleaning, Disinfection, and Sterilization Techniques for Implant Abutments

Hamid R. Shafie

Washington Hospital Center, Department of Oral and Maxillofacial Surgery, Washington, DC; and American Institute of Implant Dentistry, Washington, DC

INTRODUCTION

Implant abutments should be cleaned, disinfected, and, in specific clinical procedures and cases, be sterilized. It is important to carefully follow all procedural instructions to avoid any liability. Effective cleaning and disinfection is essential to totally sterilize implant abutments. Prior to sterilization, implant abutments should be kept clean when being handled in the dental laboratory. It is also important to follow any legal regulations valid for your local area as well as the hygienic procedures of your dental practice. This applies particularly to the different guidelines concerning the inactivation of prions.

CLEANING, DISINFECTING, AND STERILIZING IMPLANT ABUTMENTS

Cleaning

The following steps should be following when cleaning abutments.

Step 1. Rinse the abutment under flowing water while brushing the outer and inner side with adequate brushes.

Step 2. Immerse the abutment in a compatible cleaning solution (e.g. Cidezyme/Enzol™, Johnson & Johnson). The cleaning agent or disinfectant should not contain any of the following ingredients: strong organic acids or mineral acids, strong lye, organic solvents (e.g. acetone, ether, hexane, benzin), oxidizing agents (e.g. peroxide), halogens (chlorine, iodine, bromine), or aromatic, halogenated hydrocarbons.

Step 3. Rinse the implant abutment at least three times with water.

Disinfection

Use a high-level disinfectant such as Cidex OPA™ (Johnson & Johnson) for disinfecting implant abutments.

Step 1. Soak the abutment in the disinfectant solution for the required amount of time.

Step 2. Remove the implant abutment from the disinfectant solution.

Step 3. Rinse at least three times with highly purified water.

Step 4. Air-dry and package the implant abutment immediately.

Packaging the abutment in the dental laboratory

Insert the cleaned and disinfected implant abutment in a single-use sterilization package that fulfills the following requirements (one implant abutment per package).

* Requirements specified by regulation EN ISO/ANSI AAMI ISO 11607 should be followed.
* The packaging should be suitable for steam sterilization.
* The packaging should adequately protect the implant abutment from mechanical damage.

Sterilization

If no sterilization device is available in the laboratory, proper sterilization should occur at the dental office. Recommended procedures should be followed for the sterilization of implant abutments.

Reusability

You may only sterilize the abutment once. In case of inadvertent contamination, you may re-sterilize once after cleaning and disinfection.

Steam Sterilization

The following requirements should be fulfilled.

* Fractionated vacuum or gravity procedures (with sufficient product drying) should be followed.
* The steam sterilizer should fulfill ISO 17665: 2006 or EN 13060 and EN 285 requirements or equivalent national standards.
* The steam sterilizer should be validated according to EN ISO/ANSI AAMI 17665 (previously EN 554/ ANSI AAMI ISO 11134) commissioning and product specific performance qualifications.
* Sterilization time should be 20 minutes at 121°C or 3 minutes at 132°C.

CLEANING AND STERILIZING ABUTMENT ADJUSTMENT INSTRUMENTS

It is crucial that all of the instruments are properly maintained, cleaned, and sterilized after each use. All infection control principles should be applied during the cleaning and sterilization steps. A proper maintenance protocol insures the maximum effective life of the instrument.

Cleaning

The following steps should be followed.

Step 1. Inspect each instrument for any kind of damage including, but not limited to:
* Excessive wear and tear.
* Visible notches at the corners and edges.
* Distortion in the shape of polishing rubbers/silicones or the shaft of any of the instruments. This is a concern with long and narrow instruments.

   Note: Always wear gloves when handling a contaminated instrument. A brand new instrument should replace any instrument that fails to pass the visual inspection step.

Step 2. Use an ultrasonic unit and general purpose cleaning solution to loosen large debris on the surface of the instruments. Leave the instruments in the ultrasonic unit for 10 minutes. Rinse all the instruments under running water and use a bur brush to remove any residual debris.

   Note: Do not use aggressive cleaning solutions, such as hydroclic acid-based types, as they may corrode the instruments. Prolonged ultrasonic steps may cause the instrument color code to come off.

Step 3. Use paper towels to dry all of the instruments, ready for the sterilization step.

Sterilization

To eliminate any cross-contamination from patient to patient or from patient to lab technician and/or dentist, all of the instruments *must* be sterilized after each use. There are three methods for the sterilization of instruments: dry heat, steam autoclave, and cold sterilization.

Dry Heat

If you are using a dry heat sterilizer, the following steps should be completed.

Step 1. In order to transport the instruments into the dry heat sterilizer, use one of the following methods:
* Wrap the instruments using foil, double-layered cotton, or muslin fabric.
* Put unwrapped instruments on a tray.
* Place the instruments and other items in a lidded metal container.

Step 2. Place the instruments in the oven and heat to the designated temperature. The oven must have a thermometer or temperature gauge to make sure the designated temperature is reached. Use the list in the box to determine the appropriate amount of time to sterilize instruments at different temperatures (do not begin timing until the oven reaches the desired temperature, and do not open the oven door to add or remove any items). The times shown represent the amount of time that items must be kept at the desired temperature to insure sterilization is achieved. Keep in mind that the total cycle time – including heating the oven to the correct temperature, sterilization, and cooling – is usually twice as long as the time noted here.

Note: Because dry heat can dull sharp instruments, carbide burs should not be sterilized at temperatures higher than 160°C.

Sterilization times at different temperatures

- 170°C (340°F): 1 hour
- 160°C (320°F): 2 hours
- 150°C (300°F): 2.5 hours
- 140°C (285°F): 3 hours

Step 3. Leave the instruments in the sterilizer to cool before removing. When they are cool, remove items using a sterile pick-up and use or store immediately.

Step 4. Store the instruments properly. Proper storage is as important as the sterilization process itself:

- *Wrapped instruments:* Under optimal storage conditions and with minimal handling, properly wrapped instruments can be considered sterile as long as the wrappings remain intact and dry. For optimal storage, place sterile packs in closed cabinets. When in doubt about the sterility of a pack, consider it contaminated and re-sterilize it.
- *Unwrapped instruments:* Use unwrapped instruments immediately after removal from the sterilizer or keep them in a covered, clean, uncontaminated container.

Steam Autoclave

If you are using a steam autoclave, complete the following steps.

Step 1. Avoid arranging the instruments together tightly because this prevents steam from reaching all the surfaces.

Step 2. Either wrap the instruments or place them in a perforated container.

Step 3. Because there are many types of autoclaves in use around the world, it is difficult to provide guidance on the specific instructions of operating each one. Follow the manufacturer's instructions whenever possible. In general, sterilize wrapped instruments for 30 minutes and unwrapped instruments for 20 minutes at 121°C and 106 kPa pressure.

Note: The units of pressure marked on an autoclave's pressure gauge may vary from one autoclave to another. The box lists the correct level of pressure for autoclaving in different units (which are approximately equivalent).

Autoclaving pressure in different units

- 15 lb/in^2 (15 pounds of force per square inch)
- 106 kPa (106 kilopascals)
- 1 atm (1 atmosphere)
- 1 kgf/cm^2 (1 kilogram of force per square centimeter)
- 776 torr
- 776 mmHg (776 millimeters of mercury)

Because of the potential for corrosion, autoclaving carbide instruments can reduce the life of the instruments.

Cold Sterilization

Most chemical/cold sterilization solutions render instruments sterile only after 10 hours of immersion. This prolonged chemical action can be more detrimental to carbide instruments than the usual 20-minute autoclave cycle. If instruments need to be *disinfected* only, a chemical/cold sterilization soak is acceptable. Generally, disinfection will take approximately 10 minutes or more. Check the manufacturer's specifications.

Note: Keep in mind the difference between sterilization and disinfection. Since cold sterilizers contain an oxidizing agent, it is not recommended to cold sterilize carbide instruments.

REFERENCES AND ADDITIONAL READING

3M Lava. Sterilization guidelines.
GC Advanced Technologies. In office sterilization guidelines.
Jota. Sterilization guidelines.
Komet. General instructions for use and safety recommendations for the application of rotary and oscillating dental instruments.

Index

Page numbers in *italics* refer to figures.
Page numbers in **bold** refer to tables.

Clinical and Laboratory Manual of Dental Implant Abutments, First Edition. Edited by Hamid R. Shafie.
© 2014 John Wiley & Sons, Inc. Published 2014 by John Wiley & Sons, Inc.